LIVING
OUR
DYING

LIVING
OUR
DYING

A Way to the Sacred in Everyday Life

Joseph Sharp

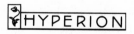

New York

Reprint permissions appear on pp. 233–234.

Book design by Elena Erber

Library of Congress Cataloging-in-Publication Data

Sharp, Joseph, 1961–
Living our dying : a way to the sacred in
everyday life / Joseph Sharp. — 1st ed.
p.   cm.
Includes bibliographical references.
ISBN 0-7868-6230-0
1. Terminally ill—Religious life.   2. Death—Religious aspects.
3. Spiritual life.   4. Sharp, Joseph, 1961–   . I. Title.
BL625.9.S466   1996
291.4'4—dc20   95-41951
CIP

First Edition
2 4 6 8 10 9 7 5 3 1

In memory of the following "fellow travelers"
along life's path who, each in their own way,
taught me the importance of coming to
live my own dying:

Craig Anderson
Ron Boyd
Irene Castloo
Bill Franklin
Kitty Gregg
Christopher W. Hancock
Stephen Hunter
Matthew Jones
Jerry Lankford
Michael Petty
Topsy Sharp
Lynn Stanford
Jeffery Wadlington
Jody Weger

And also dedicated to my partner-in-life,
Barry Day Lewis, for being the constant mirror in
which I watch myself living my own dying.

Contents

Acknowledgments ix
Before You Begin xiii
Preface: Why Bother? xv

A Sacred Paradox 1

I. WAKING UP TO OUR DYING
1. Honest Beginnings 7
Take a Moment . . . 23

II. INVITING DYING INTO EVERYDAY LIFE
Introduction 27
2. Effort, Pushing Through: Some Basic Practices 30
3. Taking Another Look 44
4. The Self That Doesn't Die 69
A Guided Meditation 88

III. GOING DEEPER
Introduction 101
5. More Stories, Reflections, and Practices 104
6. The Mirror: Being Alive with Someone
As They Die 129
7. Moment to Moment . . . and the Moment
of Death 166

IV. LIVING OUR DYING
8. Relationships 181
9. Activism 192
10. Intimacy with All Things 208

Afterword 224
Suggestions for Further Reading 229

"Follow your inner heart and the world moves in and helps," Joseph Campbell said. That's what the process of writing this book felt like. So many people helped in so many ways. Here's my list:

To begin with, I wish to acknowledge the people who've been with me now for a long time: My parents, Joe and Brenda Sharp, for their strength and support. My sister and dear friend, Lesley Sharp, for her courage and honesty. My soul-mate and partner-in-life Barry Day Lewis for pushing me to grow, confront my own fears, and for being the mirror in which I watch myself living my own dying. Guinevere Grier for her friendship and vision to see that an HIV+, non-ordained, non-seminarian could serve himself and others as an intern chaplain for AIDS patients at Parkland Memorial Hospital. Becky Evans for many things, including the laptop Macintosh I wrote this on. My aunt Martha Neil for her faith and prayers. Carl Michel for his belief in my talents and support of my life process.

And I must single out my good friend and fellow traveler Joy Williams, who continually convinced me of the value of my writings and message whenever I doubted myself. Joy, this book would probably not have come into being without your ongoing insistence that I write, write, write.

I must also acknowledge Larry Dossey, M.D., and Marianne Williamson, who have both supported my writings from the beginning. Thank you both. And thanks, Larry, for connecting me to Kitty Farmer.

And to Kitty Farmer and Ned Leavitt, both my agents and fellow travelers along the path, thank you for your guidance, artistry and expertise in leading me with such integrity and heart through the world of writing and selling a book. A writer could not be more blessed. Also thanks to Kip Kotzen for making my life easier.

Thank you to Leslie Wells, my editor, and to Bob Miller, Hyperion's publisher—both fellow living-our-dying activists—for having the personal depth and vision to see what this book is truly about. And to the entire staff at Hyperion who has worked so hard to make this book see the light of an actual bookstore, thank you as well. Also at Hyperion, I must thank Editorial Assistant Jennifer Lang; and also Victor Weaver for a cover art design that speaks more than any words could convey.

Thank you to the following authors for believing in the message of this book with such heartfelt enthusiasm that they put the considerable authority of their names behind this work: Larry Dossey, Joan Halifax, Thomas Moore, M. Scott Peck, and Marianne Williamson. (And my apologies to those of you whose endorsements arrived too late to be included on this list.)

Some of this project was first written at the HIV writing group, "Write Action," I attend in Santa Fe. I wish to thank poet Joan Logghe, who single-handedly facilitates the group. Joan, your dedication and compassion are appreciated. I also wish to thank the other "regulars" who've attended Write Action's group: Nancy Barickman, Steve Dobuszynski, Sally Fisher, Robert Levithan, Jim Rondone, Mary Shapiro, and Janet Vorhess.

I also wish to thank Tina, the nurse who allowed me to reprint portions of her private journal.

And some people who've cared for me (in many ways) as I've written this book: my therapist, a true doctor of the soul, Dorothy Rogers; my medical doctor, Trevor Hawkins, M.D., and all the nurses and staff at the clinic of the AIDS Wellness Project in Santa Fe, New Mexico; my acupuncturist and herbalist, Makima Byron; the New Mexico AIDS Services and Santa Fe Cares; Catherine Hebenstreit for her support during the book negotiation process; and Rudi Florian for the anonymous poem in the "Relationships" chapter. I also wish to thank Anthony Rippo, M.D., at the Santa Fe Institute of Medicine and Prayer; Mitchell Ivers; Theo G. Romine; Inette Miller; Marcia Tyson Kolb; Nancy Lewis; Lynn Gifford; the staff and patrons at Downtown Subscription Coffee Shop and the Santa Fe Baking Company for letting me sit and write for hours upon hours; and, finally, the city and people of Santa Fe, New Mexico, for immediately making a stranger living his dying of AIDS feel right at home. I thank and honor you all.

Before You Begin—
This Book Is Not for the "Diagnosed" Only

You need not be "diagnosed" with a terminal or life-
threatening condition to benefit from this book. You need
only to be waking up to the fact that you and those you love
are going to die one day. That's enough to begin to live
your dying—which is to live your life, too.

This book is not for the diagnosed only. It is for everyone
who finds himself or herself, here, in a body.

Why Bother?

Like a lot of baby boomers, I grew up watching television reruns of *Star Trek*. Every so often, it seemed, Spock would die and Dr. McCoy would turn to Captain Kirk, pause, and stoically announce, "He's dead, Jim." But by the end of the show Spock had always miraculously recovered, still an integral part of the crew, exploring the universe day after day, rerun after rerun. After all, he was one of the principal characters. And we all knew that the principals never really died—only extras and guests could die. Everyone knew that the stars of the show lived forever.

It was a shock to find out *Star Trek* was lying to me all those years. I'd come to believe death wasn't real. It couldn't happen and when it did, it was always a mistake, corrected before the final bow. I believed death could never happen to me or anyone else who had one of those coveted starring roles in my drama. Only the extras and guest stars, remember. Not me. Not the principals of my show. I think a lot of us believed that when we were younger. The stars of our show would live forever.

Years later, into adulthood, we found out otherwise. For me, it was AIDS. I woke up from my dream of immortality to find many of the stars in my drama dying—and they never miraculously returned in the next scene. For you, perhaps it will be AIDS too, or leukemia or heart disease or some kind of cancer or perhaps a sudden accident. The possibilities are almost limitless. And if it isn't you or me who is suddenly dying, it will be our parents, our friends, our immediate family, or even our children. Upon that awakening it will seem as if death is, almost magically, everywhere we look. Yesterday death was something unreal that only happened around the periphery of life; today it's as intimate as our own breath.

Back in 1984, I knew I was sick. I just didn't feel right inside. Friends were dying of AIDS, but I didn't really let it affect me. Even when I was given a prognosis of three years to live, I still denied the whole thing. After all, my disease was not so airtight. It was new, unpredictable. The medical authorities might be wrong, I told myself. (And as it turned out, they were wrong about my three years; it's now been over ten years since that diagnosis.) But my "beating the odds" and becoming a long-term survivor was no lasting satisfaction, because something else lingered. Though the prognosis in time was wrong, the basic truth of "Joseph, you are going to die" lingered. That truth is really what I was running from. I didn't want to hear about that. I wanted to get on with my life as it was before. I had too many things to do, I thought. I was, to put it simply, in denial of my dying process.

Most of us are. Why shouldn't we be? Why would any of us consciously choose to embrace and feel the pain of our life's impermanence, of our dying? This is an important question. Why should we take the time and energy to do the emotional and spiritual work of consciously living our dying? Why bother?

About that, the Indian mystic and poet Kabir says:

Friend, hope for the [truth] while you are alive.
Jump into experience while you are alive! . . .
What you call "salvation" belongs to the time before
*   death.*

If you don't break your ropes while you are alive,
do you think
ghosts will do it after?

The idea that the soul will join with the ecstatic
just because the body is rotten—
that is all fantasy.
What is found now is found then.
If you find nothing now,
you will simply end up with an empty apartment in the City
*   of Death.*
If you make love with the divine now, in the next life
*   you will have the face of satisfied desire.*

So plunge into the truth, find out who the Teacher is,
*   Believe in the Great Sound!*

But I can speak only for myself. I've come to find that if I don't live my dying, I'm not honestly living my life's whole-ness. There's a separation—a compartmentalization, an incompleteness—to my present life experience if I close

myself off from my dying. This closing off is not just intellectual; it is mostly a feeling. I feel myself closed and separated
from life, from myself and others, from God. Such a separate
life is no longer enough. I need to experience my life as a
whole, not just the sanitized parts. And like Kabir in his
poem, I need to experience that wholeness now, not just
later in something called "heaven." This is my journey.

Where is whole life to be found? Jesus taught that
the kingdom of God was within us, and to emphasize how
intimately present this kingdom was he proclaimed it to
be "at hand"—right here, right now. Buddha taught the
same. Both our suffering and enlightenment are in this very
experience of the here and now. These teachers each asked
in their own way, "If not here and now, where else will we
find the whole life?" I bother to live my dying because I
want to experience the whole life in this life.

Dying is inseparable from living. Two sides of one
whole coin. Most of us in this culture spend the majority
of our lives actively denying that dying side of the coin.
This book is a plea for us to stop this denial. It is a plea
for you and me, collectively and individually, to open our
hearts and minds to all of life, which must include our
dying. From personal experience with my own terminal
illness, I know that once a person consciously begins this
process of opening to his or her dying, life begins to radically
change. A spiritual and emotional acceleration occurs. An
awakening begins. And this awakening happens regardless
of one's religious preference or spiritual tradition. (Try
thinking of our varied spiritual traditions not as different
beliefs, but as the different languages and metaphors in
which humankind tries to imagine the One Unimaginable

Reality of God. What they each speak of and direct us toward is the Same One Reality.) My hope is that the stories, practices, and suggestions in this book will help you progress along your chosen spiritual path in whatever form that takes. No religion has a monopoly on living the whole life or on truth.

So at this point in my journey, I can no longer keep my dying away. Disguising it, calling it by another name, denying it—none of this works any more. If I am going to live, and I mean really live with all the zest and authenticity of life, I am going to have to fully embrace my dying, too.

Living my dying certainly isn't always pleasant or comfortable.

And I still resist and want to quit from time to time.

Nevertheless, I feel myself changing, opening. I'm no expert. I'm just a student like you. The reflections, stories, and practices contained in this book are notes of my personal experience. I hope they help.

So I bother to live my dying because it is my way to live a truly honest and whole experience in this life. To me it is a way to the Sacred in everyday life.

My prayer is that you bother too.

And you don't need to be officially diagnosed with a life-threatening illness to bother. You just need to wake up to the fact that your body is going to die one day and there must be more to life than what you're currently experiencing. That's enough to begin this book. That's enough to begin to live your dying—which is to live your life, too.

Joseph Sharp

Santa Fe, New Mexico

A Sacred Paradox

I remember the first time someone asked me to assist her in dying. She was a mother in her late forties, with a wide round beautiful face that was not uncommon for the rural people of northeast Texas. Though she was on a morphine drip and not, in her own words, "in too much pain," the tumors in her had grown to such a size that they pressed against her spinal column, paralyzing her from the upper chest down. Almost every function of life had to be performed for her. She couldn't urinate or defecate for herself, or even press the buzzer to call a nurse. Her doctors didn't know how much longer she would live, perhaps another week, perhaps a bit more or a lot less. It could be a withering, slow death.

When I walked into the hospital room, her husband put his chin to his chest, shook my hand, and excused himself without looking me directly in the eyes. He left the room, glancing down to the floor. A teenage daughter was also present and though there were tears in her eyes, she was smiling. "I'll be outside," she said. "Momma wants to be alone with you."

As I moved bedside, I noticed the glow you sometimes see around those who are in the final stages of their dying process. "Hello, my name's Joseph. I'm the chaplain. The head nurse said you wanted to talk to me." The wide thick face softened more as she smiled. Her eyes glistened.

It was as if she reached out her hands and gave me a long, slow embrace, as sweet and thick and moist as those east Texas summers she had lived her whole life through. But of course only her face had moved. Everything else was still. "Yes, Honey, I wanted to see you. They told me you do other things than just regular preaching and praying."

She watched me closely. I nodded, not quite sure what she was getting at. The woman tilted her head toward the bedside table. I saw a copy of Bernie Siegel's book Love, Medicine and Miracles. "I've been doing the kind of things that Doctor Siegel said to do. Visualizations an' such. I think they helped some, but they didn't cure me. I'm not in too much pain right now, but sometimes it gets real bad. They don't know how much longer I've got." She smiled and closed her eyes for a moment. She seemed to float off somewhere for a few seconds but then was back, eyes shining at me. "I'd like to know if you'll help me do something?"

"Of course," I said softly. "Anything."

"Well, I'd like for you to do a visualization for me. I want you to help me go ahead an' die. Can you do that, Honey? Can you do me a visualization where I just go into God's arms an' don't come back?"

I felt my stomach grab and my breath stop. At that moment it was clear to me that everyone else in her family knew what was happening. They'd paid their last respects and had been waiting for me to arrive and do what Momma wanted.

There are no words that can begin to convey how, in that moment, my heart broke at her pain, at my own pain, at the whole world's pain. Or, at how, in that same intolerably painful moment, God was also right there in all His grace and strength. And I felt a tingling of fear, but a good fear, a grounding, humbling fear—truthfully, an awe at this very moment. A sacred paradox. Her eyes shimmered, vibrant black dots of total aliveness and invitation. "Will you, Honey?"

I spoke carefully and slowly, "Yes, I can try."

She closed her eyes and the gentle smile softened as her face smoothed out into a deep, peaceful sea. "Thank you. I'm ready now. Go ahead."

part I

WAKING UP TO OUR DYING

When is death not within ourselves?

—HERACLITUS

(540–480 B.C.)

chapter 1

Honest Beginnings

*In a society that is able to send a man to
the moon and bring him back well and
safe, we have never put any effort into the
definition of human death. Isn't that
peculiar?*

—ELISABETH KÜBLER-ROSS

Dying can be scary. It's one of the biggest taboos in our culture. We don't want to bring dying home to where we live, down into the bones of our daily lives. We want to keep it out. Away in the hospital. Away in the nursing home or hospice. It's something we'd rather experience through movies and television—like a painful news report we can end by switching the channel. I understand this. After all my work, dying still scares me at times, and I find myself hurriedly switching channels in my mind. This is okay. Waking up to our dying is an ongoing process. There are moments we are more awake and moments we are less. I remember a time in my life when I was so fearful I couldn't even say the word "died." But now I can say the

7

word. Now, when I'm fearful, I can even feel and say, "I'm scared." This is all part of the process of living our dying.

This book is about that process. It is not about making dying into some wondrous, mystical, or pretty thing (though our processes may at times be each of these); instead it's about honesty toward what we're experiencing. We are honest so we can open wider to experience our living and dying from a freer perspective. Living our dying is about pushing up against our boundaries around death, loosening the taboos, and inviting dying back home into the daily marrow of life. This takes a commitment to honesty. We could also say living our dying takes dedication and courage—that's true—but honesty is the ground upon which everything else stands. So in this book, we will continually come back to honesty. It is where we begin and return again and again.

We've all heard it said that "Everyone is dying from the moment they are born." But if we're honest, most of us don't really believe "I'm dying" until we near the end of our lives. Some of us never believe it, refusing to live our dying right up to the moment of death. I've also heard it said, "We will die as we live." If we lead a life of fear, for example, we'll die in fear. If we lead a life of joy and peace, we'll die in joy and peace. From my experience with dying, this is too simple. I've never known a living, breathing human being who doesn't experience some fear at least some of the time. (And I know some seemingly peaceful people who are on Prozac.) The painful truth is, there are no simple formulas. Living, dying, and death are a lifelong experience that can't be sorted out neatly with platitudes.

To begin moving into a place of mind where we can wake up to our dying, we'll need to develop a larger view of it all—of dying, living, the world, ourselves. Our problem is that most of us really want a smaller view. A smaller view helps to make life seem simple. If our perspective is narrow, so is the range of choices from which we have to choose. With a narrow perspective, we can justify statements like: "Well, death's inevitable so I'd better just live this life with as much joy and happiness as I can. And since there's no choice about it, I'm certainly not going to dwell on something as unpleasant as death and dying. That's just the way things are."

At first this statement might sound like an open acceptance of death and dying, but a closer look reveals the opposite. We've limited our view and can see no alternative but to deny the "inevitable" until it slaps us in the face. And if we're determined to experience only "joy and happiness" we will most likely miss the actual experience of our own dying—let alone those experiences with our friends and family who are dying. This is running away. The view has been established beforehand. I know. It used to be my view. In my family of origin, we didn't talk about "it." Even after my paternal grandfather died (the first of my family to die in my life), we still didn't speak of death other than to affirm occasionally how Pa was in heaven with God now. That was enough said.

Many of us see this choice of keeping dying separate from daily life as something inherent, even natural—again, "That's just the way things are." Life in one corner, death in the other. In fact, however, this view is not natural; it is cultural. This "life as separate from death" view is a product of contemporary Western, industrialized culture. Other cultures throughout our world history have seen (and still see) death and dying in a wholly different light. A friend and colleague of mine tells a story about her experiences with death and dying when she lived in India for several years:

> Every single day you see dead bodies carried openly through the streets on stretchers. Bodies are not hidden away, no coffins. People in the procession are singing, chanting, and banging drums. It's all part of everyday life, this march to the burning grounds. And often, as you're going about your daily business, you're walking in the procession too, whether you like it or not. The dead and dying are everywhere in the streets. In India they aren't whisked out of sight. So even as you do your daily shopping, you're part of this ongoing dying that's all around you. You can't escape it and wouldn't even think to try.
>
> Dying is in the home, too. Like most third-world countries, India is a place of the extended family. And there aren't many hospitals. So most people die at home. Just about everyone, as they grow up, has spent a lot of time in the company of someone who's dying. It's a natural part of life's experience.

How different from our culture, where we have been insulated and protected from death and dying. Many Westerners, even at middle age, have never spent any extended time in the presence of someone dying. And though epidemics such as AIDS have helped to open the doors that death and dying once hid behind, much of the awareness that has come still remains cloistered within the gay and healthcare communities. The fact is that mainstream America has not yet begun to let dying out of its closet. But the door has been unlocked.

Occasionally someone asks me, "What can I do to help bring a greater awareness of dying into the mainstream?" I think the best advice is: live your own dying. In our own individual, personal example is the collective world healed. We must live it for ourselves first.

In the Eastern spiritual traditions that I'm aware of, one of the basic aims of life is to prepare for death. What happened to us in the West? What happened to our Western culture and religion that we've so separated our dying from our living? The ancient Greeks, from whom our civilization sprang, kept death and dying in the center of their lives and philosophy as a constant reminder that today's life must be lived fully and ethically. Socrates himself proclaimed, "true philosophers make death and dying their profession." Why have we so diligently removed dying from our daily life?

I'm not going to try to answer this question directly. It is important for each of us to inquire into this for him- or herself.

Why have we so diligently removed dying from daily life?

Just one admonition: it is too easy to blame our culture, church, or parents. We need to go deeper than the surface political or economic reasons for why we separate dying from daily living. Deeper into our hearts and minds. We must ask ourselves sincerely: "Why do I want to live my life without the shadow of death near me? What is it I fear will happen if I'm really honest about death and dying?"

Recognizing the Cracks

We've all tried to imagine what it would be like to have a doctor give us a terminal diagnosis. There's something epic about it. It's definitely a "big scene" in our life's drama. The protective egg we have lived in all those years—the illusion of "I'll live forever"—now has a crack. The surprise for me was, when the crack happened for real, it didn't change me as much as I'd imagined it would. I am not alone in this.

For myself and many others who have been similarly diagnosed, receiving the terminal prognosis was definitely *not* the vehicle that carried us further. Most of us deny our dying. I did for years. It's a romantic ideal to think that the doctor's pronouncement of "Ah, you have only a few months or years left to live" is going to somehow change us in any *lasting* way. If only it were that easy. Even though receiving a diagnosis can be terrifying and can bring us to recognize the cracks in our fairy-tale "I'll live forever" egg, it finally won't crack the egg *open*. We have to do that for ourselves. The human mind's ability to handle and deny the terrifying is profound. It takes work and commitment to really wake up to our dying. A crack in our egg does not a newborn self make.

Clearly, a terminal diagnosis provides an impact from without. And, yes, sometimes this impact can be so powerful that it cuts through our defenses in a single blow, but even that is not enough. There must be an *inner response* to the impact. There must be an inner willingness toward *not* rebuilding our same old life-concept of "I'll live forever" again—not listening to the voice that says, "Okay, Joseph, it's time to get back into the stream of life and forget this silly dying business; you've got work to do." In my own journey with terminal illness, I've come to see that it wasn't until I truthfully started to *live* my dying on a day-to-day basis that I began to realize the preciousness of my life with any ongoing clarity. Of course, the fact that "I am going to die" was brought more immediately to my attention because of my diagnosis, but again that knowledge in itself certainly wasn't enough. And it certainly wasn't something that made me extra-special. We are all going to die, aren't we? But just accepting that fact won't get us very far, though it is a beginning.

Acceptance of our dying must become an *ongoing* action. I try to reaccept my dying daily. This is certainly more difficult than getting diagnosed. The difference is between reaccepting my own dying on a daily, moment-to-moment basis (which is a process of inner change) and just receiving the one-time blow of a terminal prognosis. The difference is between authentic growth and fear-oriented ego games.

What changes us is not the bad news, but the daily, experiential living with it. In this process we cultivate the courage and honesty to really live with our dying and not hide in denial. This is not easy. Most of our world will support us in denying our mortality. No one wants to look at your reality unless they are also willing to look at their own. As we live our dying, we begin to develop a sense of "self" that exists not in a safe little egg, but a larger, less defined Self that lives and moves and flows in a world of ongoing impermanence. You might think that someone diagnosed with terminal cancer or AIDS has it easier when it comes to realizing this larger Self. Perhaps. But also, perhaps not. It is all too tempting to compartmentalize our "disease" and "diagnosis" into something we only deal with part time. Just because I've been officially diagnosed doesn't guarantee I'll also recognize the inner diagnosis that "I'm dying even now."

It is crucial to recognize the cracks in our egoic egg. And the impact of a terminal diagnosis is some good stuff to practice with, but it's only that—the stuff of practice. Real growth comes from within. We need to develop an *inner practice* of pushing through the cracks. Living our dying puts the responsibility back upon you and me, individually, for change. "Okay, my belief that I'll live forever is actually cracked. But it is up to me to push through the cracks and open into a more spacious experience beyond this little ego-self." Living our dying asks us to practice pushing through our cracks every day.

And I think I should tell you up front that there are not any pat formulas for doing this. It is a very individual endeavor. And it is probably the most difficult thing for a human being to do. To do this is to confront our greatest fear.

The Unofficial Diagnosis

These last few years I've spent a lot of time speaking to groups around the country about my own terminal illness and how it has been one of the vehicles for my emotional and spiritual growth. Inevitably someone asks, "How can I come to seeing my life as part of my dying without first having to get cancer or AIDS or some other life-threatening disease?" Good question. How can those of us who haven't been terminally diagnosed come to the realization that we are dying too?

Let's look at that question directly. If you're not diagnosed with a life-threatening condition that is terminal, what then? One response might be, "Well, we are all dying from the moment we're born. So we are all terminally diagnosed." But if we're honest, this answer is of no lasting help. It is merely an intellectual understanding. I find it arrogant to believe that the intellectual fact that "we're all going to die one day" somehow equals the *experiential realization* of "I'm dying now." In actuality it does make a difference to have your doctor, the entire medical establishment at large, your neighbors, friends and family, the media—all of your world—agree, "Yes, you are dying now." Believe me, it's easy enough to deny one's dying even after getting a terminal diagnosis; it must be doubly easy without.

So if you are not terminally diagnosed in any official capacity, I think we can dismiss the "we're all in this terminal boat together" idea. In a higher truth, we are; but in our daily living experience, we're in different boats altogether. In daily life, one is traveling with chemotherapy, with fatigue so profound that walking to the bathroom is the morning's exercise, and with a day-to-day existence. Another is traveling with aerobic classes three times a week, a glass of wine with dinner, and talk of where to vacation next summer. Here the question returns. How can you proceed without that "official" diagnosis? Is trying to live your dying pointless without it?

Like most other parts of the journey, I think the key here is honesty. Honestly begin with: "Right now, I'm not terminally diagnosed in any official way." And with that said, begin seriously to seek for what you are diagnosed with in an "unofficial" way. We are each facing some kind of life-challenging condition in our lives. As Thoreau pointed out, most of us lead lives of quiet desperation. So the question is: Are we willing to look honestly at that condition? Some of us have come to understand that our quiet desperation is as much a life-threatening condition as cancer or AIDS. Isn't the teenager who can't find meaning in his or her existence facing a life-threatening condition? Do we need to wait until that teenager commits suicide or overdoses on drugs to admit to a problem? I see physical disease and emotional illness in a similar manner. We need not wait until the disease manifests physically to admit there is a problem. The problem has existed all along.

To recognize this is no small matter. You can't just snap your fingers and say, "Oh, I see that my life is actually filled with life-threatening challenges" and truthfully mean it. It takes work, self-discovery, and commitment to honesty. The good news is we all have a life-threatening condition if we open our hearts to life as it really is. So I think the best advice is not to con yourself with "We're all going to die anyway," but to genuinely work on the process of opening to your own very real suffering that is even now all around you, if you honestly look. Begin there, which is to say, begin right here with what's before you. You may have to do some serious and honest digging into your life.

No less than the person who has received an official diagnosis of heart disease or breast cancer, you too must begin with honesty. Explore your "unofficial" diagnosis. You'll begin to notice that there is a resonance between you and those of us who are officially diagnosed. You'll begin to experience that, though we appear to be in different boats, we are in truth upon the same sea. I don't believe you need to be officially diagnosed with a terminal illness to begin living your dying. But you do need to be waking up to the fact that you and everyone you love are going to die one day, and there must be more to life than what you're currently experiencing. That's enough to begin.

Honesty Toward Death

A friend says it casually over burgers and fries. A movie star says it on a television talk show. You might say it to yourself after reading a stirring account of someone's near-death experience. It goes something like this: "Well, I'm not really afraid of death. Actually, I'm sort of looking forward to what it'll be like. I'm really excited about it all."

Yes, we may believe it. We may even speak of it with an air of excitement. But I tell you, when we say this, usually we're lying. It may be partially true that we're "looking forward," but it's not wholly true. Everyone fabricates stories about their death and dying. The question we must ask ourselves is: "Is my story truthfully what I believe?" Let's proceed carefully . . .

To begin with, if pressed, most of us who tell stories like "I'm not afraid, but excited about death" will have to add an addendum (if we're honest). We will probably have to add, "Okay, I'm looking forward to what happens after death, but I'm not exactly looking forward to the process of dying beforehand." If pressed further, we will usually admit that the thought of dying actually scares us, especially the possibility of a long, drawn-out and painful process. This is more honest, but a problem remains: death and dying are still thought of as separate and distinct experiences with little, if no, interrelation. They are part of a life model based upon compartmentalization and separation in order to bypass feeling our basic fears—as if the unexamined life will somehow be the painless life.

But let's assume that we're a bit more centered and can honestly say, "No, I look forward to my dying as well. Whatever comes I plan to experience it fully." This is closer to the truth. Perhaps it is even a verbal and intellectual declaration of "conscious dying." Yet, still, there is a separation. In this story, dying is not personally acknowledged as part of daily life, here and now. Dying remains some time off in the future. It reminds me of something a Tibetan lama once said: "People often make the mistake of being frivolous about death and think, 'Oh well, death happens to everybody. It's not a big deal, it's natural. I'll be fine.' That's a nice theory until one is dying."

Let me give a personal example. When I was a hospital AIDS chaplain, I thought I'd pretty much come to terms with death and dying. I was HIV positive after all, a long-term survivor. I'd seen a lot of death. I'd read and studied the conscious-dying literature. I'd done workshops. I'd buried friends, spoken at memorial services, consoled loved ones. I didn't really have the hubris to say I was "excited" about death and dying, but I did believe I embraced it without fear. After all, this was a vast spiritual journey and in truth we're not mere bodies. After all, I faced my own death issues daily with every AIDS patient I saw. And I carried this certainty with me when I left the hospital and began my conscious-dying counseling in the larger community. I had been to the proverbial "there and back." After all, I was terminally diagnosed too. This was the story I told myself.

But, do you know what? I hadn't ever really been sick—compared to what I've experienced by now, that is. I had never walked out onto the front porch to pick up the morning paper and been so exhausted by the effort that I didn't know if I'd make it back inside. I'd never suddenly realized, "My God, I'm actually dying here; my body is falling apart and it's not getting better." I'd never had my doctor prescribe a host of medicines for me because I would literally die soon without them. I'd never been *grateful* for those toxic medicines like AZT or ddI (with side effects I'd once so quickly condemned), so grateful because, despite their toxicity, they were actually allowing me to regain some strength by slowing the virus' progression so I might live in this body of mine a little longer. Let me preach it clearly: I didn't have a clue as to just how fearful I could become until I actually, physically, literally started to experience my own bodily dying. My previous intellectual certainty and spiritual bravado were rubbed raw by actual experience. I discovered I had some very real work to do in regard to living my life honestly, let alone living my dying with some consciousness. With the "conscious dying" slick sophistication of my former story, I'd managed to con myself quite nicely.

Reading books was one thing. Being with patients while they died was one thing. Being with friends dying was closer to home. But actually feeling myself dying was altogether another experience. Mine was such a nice story until I began feeling *my* dying for myself.

From all this I've learned that no matter how much work we've done on ourselves, we never have "death and dying" down pat. Being honest about our dying isn't comfortable. So I think it's arrogance to proclaim excitement about death and dying without accepting our other emotions as well. Excitement alone isn't wholly honest.

In her book, *Writing Down the Bones*, Natalie Goldberg tells a wonderful story about Zen Master Suzuki Roshi's dying:

> He died of cancer in 1971. When Zen masters die we like to think they will say something very inspiring as they are about to bite the Big Emptiness, something like "Hi-ho Silver!" or "Remember to wake up" or "Life is everlasting." Right before Suzuki Roshi's death, Katagiri Roshi, an old friend, visited him. Katagiri stood by the bedside; Suzuki looked up and said, "I don't want to die." That simple. He was who he was and said plainly what he felt in the moment. Katagiri bowed. "Thank you for your great effort."

And there it is. That simple. Self-honesty. It takes great effort to be self-honest in our dying. But we must, or we'll be off on the wheel of denial and false excitement. We must learn to make the room within ourselves where we can realize the utter simplicity of saying what we feel—"I don't want to die"—even as we die. We touch that honesty not in self-pity or anger, but in an open acceptance of the truth of who we are in that living moment.

Most likely the person who really feels an open-ended excitement about death and dying, won't say much about it. They know that to put such a feeling into words immediately turns it into a lie. It's like enlightenment. The person who tells us he's enlightened, most likely isn't. For truth, we look at how a person lives, not what he or she says. For truth, we look at how we live our dying. There is no shame in not wanting to die, if that's your truth. Just as there is no shame in wanting to die. No formulas, just openness, honesty, and acceptance of who we are in the moment at hand. This is the work of living our dying.

A Way to the Sacred

Many of us are coming to realize that if we are going to work sincerely on ourselves spiritually in this life, we must also work on our fears and issues regarding death and dying. This book is subtitled *A Way to the Sacred in Everyday Life*. I believe that living our dying is nothing less than a journey into the sacred, here and now. Some of us come to our spiritual quest first, realizing along the way that we must embrace dying. And some come to dying first, realizing along the way that we must embrace our spiritual journey. But this is merely the appearance of things in time. At its core, "living our dying" and "living our search for the sacred" are one journey, one experience.

What is the sacred? Shelves of books have been written about this question alone. For our purposes, let's say that the sacred is "God manifested in our life experience." It's important to remember, however, that this is only a working definition. The fourteenth-century Christian mystic Meister Eckhart said, "Whoever perceives something in God and attaches thereby some name to him, that is not God. God is ineffable." And as the great Christian apologist of this century, C. S. Lewis, proclaimed, "Not my idea of God, but God." Though some of us may know God intimately in what may be described as "a personal relationship," and some may believe in a theology that spells out clearly some of God's dos and don'ts—if we're honest to that deep indwelling presence within, I think we each realize there's a vast reservoir of God that remains unknown to us. Not our idea of God, but God the Ineffable. It is my prayer that we can come to celebrate this mystery instead of fear it. And I think the same is true for the sacred. We can't pigeonhole the sacred, as God's manifestation in life, any more than we can pigeonhole God.

Can anyone seriously ask: "What does the Holy Mystery look like?" I think not, and the reason is simple. The Holy Mystery doesn't look like any *thing*. It arises everywhere and anywhere: in the hospital room, the forest, the temple, the coffee shop, the bedroom, the funeral pyre. This experience of the Mystery arising into our awareness has much more to do with an inner event than an outer appearance. As Jesus said, the Kingdom of God is within us. So this book is about a way that seeks within ourselves too. Our fuel for this journey is "living our dying."

A Brief Note on Waking Up

It is important to understand that awakening to our dying is an ongoing process. The most honest way I've found to speak of this process is to speak of a "gradual awakening." We awaken a bit, then forget and fall momentarily back into sleep; we awaken more; and gradually, our times of wakefulness are longer and longer, and our times of sleep grow less and less.

Waking up simply means you become aware of your own and everyone else's dying process. It's a crack in the egoic egg, a conscious beginning of a journey that, in truth, began long ago.

T ake a moment and think about the time someone you felt close to died. If this was a time of intense grief, try not to dwell on that aspect for now. Try to remember the larger experience. Think of what your life was like the day or two just following the death . . .

There you are, in your usual routine of life, perhaps at work, perhaps at home, perhaps walking down a street you walk every other day. But none of it *feels* the way it usually does . . .

Remember that feeling . . .

Life has a different texture to it. Outwardly, our world goes along just as it did before. But inwardly, something has been jarred, shaken. Someone we cared about is dead. Gone. And now life doesn't make as much sense as it did yesterday.

Perhaps we consciously ask, "Why am I here? What is my purpose in life? All around me, I see it: people are born, they age, get diseases, suffer in pain, and then, they die. So, why am I here?" In our sincerely asking, sincerely experiencing the big questions, we feel a connection that shines a different light upon everything: our jobs, our relationships, family, and friends. This time is intensely personal. It can't be shared with anyone, yet it encompasses all our lives. It cannot be bound or located or pinpointed. It is everywhere, within everything.

We might think of this difference as "a sudden ability to hear." In these times, we hear a call to something bigger than our usual, small lives. This call is something clearer than the voice of our preoccupied, busy mind. It is closer to our essential being than anything else. It is under our skin, underlying our every thought. It's a special time. Somehow we feel connected to something greater.

And we may even realize that this greater awareness has always been there, beneath every moment of our life. *But we feel it now.* It is important, truly important, as if nothing else ever were. It is a call to open into the bigger experience of the bigger questions.

It is a call to wake up to our dying.

part II

INVITING DYING INTO EVERYDAY LIFE

Remember, friends, as you pass by

as you are now, so once was I.

As I am now, so you must be.

Prepare yourself to follow me.

—HEADSTONE INSCRIPTION

IN ASHBY, MASSACHUSETTS

Introduction

I n the modernized Western world, we spend much of our lives in preparation. We send our children to schools preparing them to become productive, educated members of society; we invest in Social Security, IRAs, and insurance portfolios in preparation for old age or unexpected illness; one of the largest areas of our national budget is spent in preparation for war and defense. We are a society that believes in preparation—"Be prepared," as the Boy Scouts of America motto goes. But ask someone if they've prepared for dying and most likely any response will be in terms of wills, insurance, and burial plots. Ask if there has been any deeper preparation, such as emotional work or serious spiritual seeking and, usually, we'll be answered with silence. As far as the history of humankind, this is a particularly recent occurrence. From the Egyptians to the Middle Ages, the emotional soul-centered preparation for death and dying was an integral part of becoming a man or woman.

Each spiritual or cultural tradition has its own ways and practices for preparing for death and dying. The Native Americans cultivate fearlessness and awareness of death with a death chant, practiced throughout their adult lives. Hindu and Buddhist traditions offer daily practices of meditation, chanting, and powerful mantras. The early Egyptians studied and recited chapters from their *Book of the Dead*. Similarly, Tibetans study, recite, memorize, and perform detailed spiritual practices as outlined in their own dying guidebook, the *Tibetan Book of the Dead*.

Notice that these practices in preparation for dying differ somewhat from culture to culture. Each tradition develops and cultivates its own specific methods that are applicable to its own particular cultural "personality." For example, a nomadic tribal culture like the American Indian would require a different kind of practice than city-state builders like the early Greeks. There is a lesson for us in this diversity. We have no precedent for the culture that is developing in today's rapidly changing computerized information age. Indeed, we can look to other historical peoples for guidance, but we must also recognize that we do not live in nineteenth-century Tibet nor the open planes of preindustrial America. And we are not so culturally homogeneous or well defined as our predecessors. The "melting pot" of our origins has become a fiery crucible whose contents are metamorphosing into a wholly new and unprecedented alchemical soup. It's no surprise that our spiritual life has not kept stride with our cultural evolution. In this time of changing millennia, our Western culture must discover and create practices to prepare for death and dying that are practical and workable in its uniquely modernized society.

We are talking about the importance of recognizing levels of consciousness and reality beyond the material, physical, and even psychological worlds. We are talking about making room for the Divine Mystery and Greater Process to live and breathe at the very center of our daily mechanized lives. As the novelist and philosopher André Malraux remarked, "The twenty-first century will be religious or it will not be at all." We might understand Malraux's sense of the religious as a personal sacredness that can arise within each of us and become manifest in our everyday lives. I believe we can't awaken that sacredness without opening to our individual and collective dying. When we close the door to our dying, we close the door to God's indwelling spirit as well. In this way the journey into the sacred is also the journey of going even deeper into the underworlds of fear that surround our issues with death and dying. It is through this depth of exploration that we may come to understand Teilhard de Chardin's claim: "Nothing here below is profane for those who know how to see. On the contrary everything is sacred." This is the way of living our dying in everyday life.

How do we begin to prepare? As pointed out in Chapter 1, we must begin with honesty. And we must also begin with some guidance from those who've traveled ahead of us for a while.

We begin with willingness.

We begin with ourselves.

Effort, Pushing Through:
Some Basic Practices

*Thus men will lie on their backs, talking
about the fall of man, and never make
an effort to get up.*

—HENRY DAVID THOREAU

For a three-month semester in 1990, I interned as a chaplain at Parkland Memorial Hospital in Dallas, Texas. I'd never been a chaplain before and, unlike the other interns, wasn't ordained or enrolled in seminary. I had been asked to take part in the chaplaincy program solely because of my work with a local AIDS support group called the Healing Circle. At that time in my journey, I'd only known a few people who had actually died and had never been intimately involved in someone's dying process. I knew my stint at Parkland would change that. My assigned unit was the ninth floor, east wing—the infectious disease unit, mostly an AIDS ward. There I'd see AIDS beyond the incense-burning, candle-lit, New Age music–filled environment of the Healing Circle. Every day I'd come face to face with people dying of the same disease that was growing inside of me. No place to hide.

My first day began at 8:00 a.m. with the night duty chaplains briefing those of us on the day staff about the evening's events: a multiple-vehicle accident in the E.R., two deaths, one coma; a stabbing death; a crack baby in the Pediatric I.C.U. that wasn't expected to live the day; and so forth. The business of chaplaincy at an acute-care hospital like Parkland. I didn't know what most of the initials—ICU, PICU, BICU, NICU, CICU, etc.— meant. But that was okay. Why would I? I was new to all this. When the briefing ended, everyone dispersed, leaving to begin patient rounds on their floors. I don't remember what I did for that first morning, but I didn't go up to the ninth floor. I wasn't ready for that deep of a dive. I needed some more guidance, some instruction on how to handle all this death and dying. After all, this was only my first day.

That afternoon the interns met for our first "interpersonal relations" group session. Not counting the supervising therapist, there were eight of us in the group—half new interns, half well seasoned. The session began casually with the interns from last semester joking about how this room was bigger than the previous year's, how the chairs were more comfortable. The lack of formal beginning, the supervising therapist just letting the group dynamics flow in whatever direction, made me uneasy. I sat quietly, crossing and uncrossing my legs. One of the experienced chaplains, a red-haired man with a mustache, was laughing aloud about something, when the new intern sitting on my left, almost wrenched herself out of her chair. She blurted, "I've got to say something now!"

And for a frozen split-second in time, the room was absolutely still.

"Today was my first day." The new intern spoke softly now. "This morning a patient on my floor . . . passed away."

Without hesitating further, this freshly initiated chaplain filled the room with her morning's experience, stammering about how she'd been overwhelmed but kept her calm, even though she didn't know what to do or say, even though she had to call one of the senior chaplains for help with the paperwork, and even though her hands were secretly shaking throughout the whole experience. She confessed she'd felt lost, over her head, and wanted to know what else she could have done. What else could she have said to the woman's husband? Or to the two surviving sisters? Her fist pressed into the chair's wooden armrest. "What else?"

Each of us beginners waited for a response from our supervising therapist. "This will be our first real instruction on how to deal with the difficulties of death and dying," I thought. "This will be good, this is why I'm here." I listened closely. All the therapist said, before directing the group onward, was this: "It is important not to keep your issues with death obscured. So we don't use euphemisms here. We don't say, 'passed away.' We say, 'he or she died.' Because that's what happened. Someone *died* on your floor this morning."

Practice

We are all dying. But we all don't admit it. Can you imagine what the world would be like if, just for one day, we all remembered we were dying? Can you imagine how much our life and world would change if we actually lived with the conscious awareness of our own dying, of our loved one's dying, of everyone and everything's daily dying?

To move into a larger awareness of living our dying takes effort and practice. The intellectual understanding that we must broaden our life view to include dying is a beginning, but it won't assist us much in actual day-to-day experience. We need help beyond ideas and theory. If there's no real application to everyday life and no real practice to assist us in changing, all the great ideas in the world are just that—ideas. So, before we go any deeper into this exploration of living our dying, it is beneficial to touch upon some basic practices that are designed to help us push through and into our hidden issues of death. These basic practices are each incendiary in their own way, igniting our fears to reveal the defenses that guard our closed doors. Each will bring up resistance and fear. This is good. Experiencing this kind of revelation is the point of each practice.

You may choose to read these practices casually, letting them gently work their way into your life. Or you may wish to start trying to practice one or more of these actively today. But first, just a few reminders about practice:

- Don't "should" yourself. An atmosphere of exploration and discovery is best. Remember, any psychological or spiritual practice is merely a tool for digging. It is a lens to clarify the hidden. A practice is not a goal in itself. When you forget to do a practice or don't carry through with it (implied: as you "should"), your time was not misspent. Quite often it is what we avoid or don't do in our practicing that can be most revealing about our personal areas of closure and fear. The point of practice is to bring into conscious awareness the areas where we step back from honesty, wholeness, and openness. Try not to get caught in the trap of thinking that practice is something to keep score of.

- In truth, it is not the practice itself that heals, but your intention behind the practice. If you honestly want understanding, insight, and healing, and you practice sincerely, with an inquisitive, noncondemning outlook, nothing else is required.

- Make these practices your own. If the words or images suggested in this book don't resonate with you, find those that do. Also, as you work with a practice, feel free to experiment. Play. Create.

These are tools. Use them if you can. Not all tools will work as well for all people.

Using the "D" Words

It is important to examine how we speak. Our words often betray hidden stashes of denial and avoidance. I was comfortable with my euphemisms for death and dying. In the Methodist church my parents took me to as a child, we said "passed away" or "passed over." And in the contemporary pop-healing lingo, we would say that someone made their "transition." Whatever the term, it's just poetic license for the basic fact that human beings die.

But the question many people ask, including the intern chaplain who'd been corrected that first morning of her internship, is: "Well, since I *know* that people die, why must I be so harsh and literal with my words? Especially when it just makes everyone else uncomfortable?" Or to put it another way, why must we say and think "she died" instead of something more pleasant? To begin with, using the "d" words is a practice of *undoing*. Part of the work in living our dying is to undo our hidden compartments where death issues hibernate undisturbed. This undoing takes time. So we begin with "she died" and return to this literal impermanence daily. There is an important grounding in owning the fact of worldly impermanence. If you actually practice using only the "d" words, you'll see what I mean. Try it.

A basic practice is to notice your use of euphemisms for "death" or "dying" and to begin replacing those euphemisms with the actual "d" words. When I first started this practice it was rough going. I eventually had to just stop myself in mid-sentence—like, "I remember when my grandfather passed awa . . ."—and, after taking a slow breath, correct myself aloud—" . . . when my grandfather died." It was embarrassing. Most of the time it felt harsh to make that correction publicly. But who was I really protecting from that harsh reality? The public or myself? The closer I looked at the issue, the more I realized I didn't want to face, on a very subtle level, the fact that death really happens. So I kept practicing.

Make a conscious effort to use the "d" words and notice your feelings. Are you embarrassed? How does your body react to the word? Does it contract or tighten in a particular place? For me, I'd always drop the volume of the "d" word a notch or two, sometimes to almost a whisper, like I was having to say the word "masturbation" in the same room with my mother. Notice yourself. It's a simple but profound practice. Notice, but don't condemn. The point isn't to be clinically correct, but to be self-aware.

Also, now that I've done this practice so often and worked with death and dying all these years, you might think that I'm free to go back to nicer, safer euphemisms, right? Just recently, in speaking of the recent death of a friend, I found myself fumbling over the euphemism "laying the body aside"—and, through noticing my bodily contractions and fumbled speech, I realized I was using the euphemism to avoid some of the pain caused by my friend's death. So we're always having to return to this basic practice of using the "d" words instead of euphemisms. Or, at least, I certainly am.

Seeing Change, Seeing Dying

In the following practice you are asked to train your mind to begin equating *change* and *dying* as the very same process. It is a form of "labeling" your perceptions. When you recognize change occurring—for instance, a green leaf starts to turn yellow—you mentally label that change as "dying." Of course, a change in seasons is obvious. Look too for the less obvious, the more everyday and mundane. Moving from one home to another becomes a dying process; you pack your belongings, perhaps mourn and grieve in leaving the old home, then let go to embrace the new. Relationship changes become the dying of expectations, prejudices, hopes, and desires. Progression through school, graduating from one grade to the next, becomes a series of small deaths. The same is true for career growth and work. Rites of passage such as birthdays, bar mitzvahs, baptisms, weddings, anniversaries—each can also be seen as moments of dying, death, and a movement into a greater experience of life and self. Start noting all the changes that occur in your daily experience and try seeing them as a part of a larger dying process. Think about it—even the daily brushing of your teeth is a form of dying: your sleep time has passed away; the bacteria growing on your teeth at night dies as you brush and gargle; your thoughts and plans for the day are rising and falling all the while, rising, falling, being born, dying. All of this is a vast process of dying and, of course, rebirth. But for now, we concentrate on the dying. Why? This practice asks us to train our mind to recognize all change as a dying process, partially to crack open our preconceived ideas about just what is and isn't dying. It helps to expand the view of our world and life.

Some Buddhist monks are trained in a meditation practice in which they sit at the funeral grounds and meditate on the decaying process of a corpse. (In their tradition, bodies are often not buried, but left out to be picked clean by the animals and elements—a much more environmentally correct position than we practice in the West, since everything is recycled.) The purpose of this particular meditation practice is not to harden the monks to the experience of death, but to teach them to recognize the basic impermanence of all things. What was once a living breathing person is now food for animals and insects. The body and all material things change. It's a straightforward intellectual concept. Yet only when this understanding of life's impermanence is truly taken to heart, received into daily experiential life, do we begin to see that, in fact, the burial yard is in front of us *everywhere* we look. We see change/dying everywhere as the universal constant of earthly life.

This is a big leap to make. It is part of awakened perception: the illusion of permanence is lifted and the ever-changing/dying nature of the universe revealed. The game suddenly gets much bigger.

But, let's be practical. If we are serious about meditation, wonderful. Our practice and effort will bring great results. But what if we don't really meditate? How many of us who live in this Western culture are called to become Buddhist monks? How can we begin a serious practice of seeing dying everywhere in a gradual, gentle way? I think this practice of seeing change and dying as one process is a beginning. "Seeing change, seeing dying" practice is an interactive meditation with the world. I cannot emphasize its importance enough; try it.

Taking the Occasion to Imagine Yourself Dying
A common guided meditation done at conscious-dying workshops is imagining, or visualizing, your own death. It is a good practice, but I have found that timing and occasion can make a powerful difference in this type of work. In other words, it is one thing to visualize and try to imagine or feel your own dying in a workshop environment; but it is very much another to "take the occasion"—for example, when you are sick in bed with the flu, or lonely, or sad—

and *from that space and environment* to visualize your own dying. To take the occasion from your actual daily life, and integrate a visualization/exploration of your dying into that occasion, can put some sharp teeth into the imaginative process.

It can be as simple as waking one morning, tired and groggy, and from that space, take the occasion. Lie still and let your mind begin to imagine that you're dying. Perhaps imagine that you have advanced terminal cancer and can't leave the bed without assistance. Try to imagine what it would be like, what your feelings are. Try to *feel* the texture of your life in that moment. Imagine what the rest of your day would be like. Explore your feelings.

Or perhaps you have a cold (or whatever) and are at home ill. Again, whether lying on the couch or in bed, try to imagine yourself dying. Use the particular occasion of your illness to help make the visualization seem more real. As you move around the room, getting a glass of water, taking your medicine, imagine that this sick body of yours is a dying body. Imagine the illness won't pass in a day or so, and is chronic. Open up to how those fears actually feel to you. Keep exploring.

As you work with this practice, you can imagine yourself surrendering to the dying. Opening. Accepting. You can even imagine yourself at the moment of death. Letting go.

There are no definite rules here. Experiment. One of the points of this practice is to help you develop a sense of empathy with others who are dying. Also, it begins to wear away the newness of dying as a daily experience in life. Try it. You'll find all sorts of occasions in which to imagine yourself dying. Again, experiment, create.

Turning Toward Death and Dying

The following practice of "turning toward death and dying" may also be thought of as "taking dying in." We consciously turn toward death and dying and, by doing so, invite it inside to live within our protective shell of self. So often we consciously or unconsciously turn away from dying. When a friend or family member is hospitalized, we avoid going to visit. Or if we do, we are uncomfortable and can't look anyone in the eyes. We hide from the ill and are uneasy in the company of our dying friends. The practice I am describing here is a blatant reversal of that pattern of avoidance. On the contrary, we turn to face death openly, inviting it into our everyday lives.

There are no generic instructions as to how to specifically do this practice. Make this practice your own. For some, turning toward dying may mean volunteering a few hours a week at a hospital, hospice, or nursing home. For others, it may mean becoming a "buddy" to someone who has AIDS. For a nurse or doctor in a clinical setting who encounters dying daily, turning toward dying will most likely mean something else entirely—perhaps spending more time with certain patients or asking dying patients for insights into their experience, letting these patients teach and give care instead of always being cared for. To someone else, the practice may mean visiting with an ill friend or family member. To someone terminally diagnosed, it could be joining a support group and sharing with others who are in a similar situation. And for some, turning toward death and dying begins by reading a few more books on the subject, attending a workshop, or asking friends about their experiences with death. Sometimes this turn is a dramatic confrontation, other times it's very subtle, almost unnoticeable to an outside observer. This is your own inner work, no one else's. Living our dying is an individual endeavor. No two journeys are exactly alike.

I knew a famous healer in Los Angeles who worked extensively with the AIDS and cancer communities. Yet she had a steadfast rule, "I don't do hospitals." According to her own rhetoric, she had healed her "personal issues" with death and had no further need of working in that depth. She saw such work as healing's opposite. As time passed, however, and more and more of her clients were dying in the hospital, she had to come to face what many of us in the healthcare communities have discovered: we are continually working on living our dying. We are continually turning away or toward death. The work is to become actively aware of our turnings.

Remember, there is no "should" in this practice. Try not to think, "I should be able to spend more time with my dying Grandma and shouldn't be so scared." Instead, try to cultivate a sense of exploration for the work you are capable of doing. For example, instead of "should-ing" yourself, you might ask, "I wonder why I'm so anxious to leave the hospital just after I get there? Why do I constantly feel the urge to glance away?" or "What do I feel like when I look into Grandma's eyes?" Be gentle and loving to yourself in this exploration. You are coming up against your greatest fear. This is an ongoing process and takes time.

Know that if you set hard-and-fast goals in this

practice, you will have a more difficult time dealing with your sense of fear and failure (both of which the practice is guaranteed to reveal). Though this practice is presented at the beginning of the book, it is actually a step toward one of the core practices of living our dying, that of being alive with someone as they die. (The other core practice involves being alive with yourself as you die.) Remember, this practice involves consciously *turning toward* and *inviting in* death and dying. It is *not* a question of "embracing our death and dying without blinking an eye." The goal is to be aware of yourself, your reactions, thoughts, and especially feelings as you turn toward dying. If you are like me when I began this practice, your defense mechanisms will begin to work overtime as you enter the room of someone who is dying. Fears explode into consciousness. So expect this practice essentially to involve confrontation.

Much of the emphasis of this book will be on assisting you to continue to open up in the presence of dying—your own dying and someone else's. For now, however, a spirit of willingness and exploration is all that is asked. Perhaps you can't spend much time with a loved one who is dying just yet. It may be too fearful or painful. Maybe you don't know anyone who's ill. Whatever the reason, this is okay. The practice asks only that you explore, turn toward and into, that possibility.

I can't say it enough: the practices presented here are not formulas; they are invitations to exploration. Travel guides.

Try not to use any practice to close yourself in, but to open up to a more spacious understanding. Fear and pain are part of the opening process. You are pushing up against your boundaries. Be as gentle on yourself as you can. But push on.

chapter 3

Taking Another Look

An old friend is in the hospital. He is not expected to live much longer. Though I'm a bit hesitant, I go to visit him anyway. After all, this will probably be the last time I'll see him. His impending mortality pulls at me to think about my own, something I'd rather avoid. And I've been to hospitals before. I remember the smells of urine, feces, and fresh plastic tubing that permeate the place—the smells of institutionalized dying. I haven't seen this particular friend in a while. What will he look like? Older, skinnier, balder? How ravaged will the body be? All these thoughts are my fears. But, out of some sense of responsibility or guilt, I go to the hospital anyway.

Once there, I slip quietly into his room. I force myself to smile and move to his bedside. It's only then that I notice the radiance. Being this near to him, I can even feel it. It's as if he were glowing. I see it, feel it. He seems so different. So peaceful, almost wise.

We talk, we laugh some, and he seems enlightened

in a simple, humble way. The longer I'm with him, the more I lose my sense of how much time is passing. At one point, I look at my watch and realize I've stayed for much longer than I'd planned. But it doesn't matter. I feel myself being healed in his presence. It's almost as if he is living in the next world already. There is a presence that shines through him. I feel an indescribable love flowing across to me.

And I know beyond a doubt that he *is* healed. Without hesitancy or fear, we look into each other's eyes. There is a softness between us. I would not dare to change anything. I would not dare to wish or think or pray that he be cured or changed physically in any way. I would not dare to ask that our experience be in any way other than this, now. How could I? He is moving into a peace I've never really known before. How could I wish to stop that? I'm so grateful to him. And I'm grateful that I came to the hospital. I'm so grateful for it all as he continues healing me in his sight.

Eventually, at some moment, we both know that I must be on my way. But we also know that we'll never truly part. There's no joking, no covering up our fear— because in that now-moment there is no fear remaining between us. Just openness, just spaciousness. I notice a glowing around him as I leave.

Walking down the hospital's corridor and out into the sunshine of the afternoon, I feel myself glowing too. There is such a vast openness in my heart. My friend and fellow traveler has shared his love and holy, sacred Self with me. The day is beautiful and what I call God is everywhere. I know my friend is healed. I know I am healed. It is beyond any reason. I'm just so grateful for it all.

And then, about halfway home from the hospital, the thought returns: "But he's lying there, dying."

And the gratitude slips away . . .

The awareness of perfection slips away . . .

The healing slips away . . .

And I am back into the so-called stream of life. The old world rises up before my eyes, my chest clinches, and I see only him dying . . .

What happened to me that I was able to look out upon my world and see it in such a different light? What happened that I was able to be that open? What happened— and how can I find that openness again?

Once a person starts consciously looking at his or her concerns about death and dying, the world opens up. Add to that opening some dedicated effort and practice, and serious change begins to occur. This conscious awakening into a more whole picture of life and death is actually a healing process. And like all healing processes, it takes time. But what else is time for?

During this time of opening, practice, and exploration, what we once took for granted as black-and-white will often become different shades of gray. Many of the old priorities, values, rules, and guidelines begin to shift. This too can be scary. Our world gets turned upside down. We who seek—who endeavor to live our dying—begin to think and perceive differently from those who don't. Our upside-down vision asks such questions as: "Why work so hard to get ahead in my career when it doesn't assist me in opening my heart?" Or, "What's the purpose of living if it all just ends in my dying, anyway?"

We begin to question many of our previous certainties. If we've been fixated on healing our bodies from disease, we may begin to lose interest in "winning the battle," asking questions like: "What's winning, really? Why try to beat death as if it were some enemy outside of my process?" We may even begin to see the value in statements like "turn the other cheek" or "love your enemies." We begin to understand why the Buddhists emphasize "nonattachment" to our material things (including our most material possession, our own bodies). We begin to understand what the Christians mean by "surrender." And we can no longer safely take anything we formerly believed for granted. Everything we experience is starting to look and feel different in some way. We are changing. And, like it or not, most of our world is threatened by this change.

From here we can see the wisdom of humility. This is not the time to preach "truth," but to quietly observe our lives from this newly emerging perspective. As we travel this journey, we find ourselves taking another look. This is a holy act. It is a Gift of great importance. Try not to forget that taking another look is a holy endeavor.

So I honor you for taking another look, for this new perception. Be gentle with yourself as you grow and emerge into this new perception. Again, it's a healing process and it takes time. Time is for just that, taking another look, healing—all of which is coming to know the sacred Self within you.

Healing Versus Dying

It was during my work with the Healing Circle in Dallas that I began to question the way I looked at healing versus dying. I'd been facilitating our healing group for a couple of months. Between thirty and seventy people attended each week. Maybe two-thirds were diagnosed with HIV or AIDS. The other third included everything from leukemia to loneliness. We'd begun the group in the height of the New Age self-healing movement and used many of its principles and tools: speaking only in positive terms, declaring how "perfect, whole, and complete" we each already were, doing guided visualizations and meditations, and teaching that "all forms of physical disease are outward manifestations of inner thoughts." I knew that my thoughts affected my body to some extent; I'd experienced that firsthand. So it wasn't too far-fetched for me to make the leap from the hopelessness of traditional medicine ("you've got three years to live, Joseph, and there's nothing we can do") to the positivism of the New Age movement ("there are no 100% fatal diseases; all diseases are just an outward manifestation of an inner thought, and a thought can be changed"). I believed I'd found "The Answer." Salvation was at hand, and the key was within my own mind. So desperate was my need not to die, I embraced this reasoning without hesitation or question. I needed some control over my life, and New Age positivism provided me with just that. To hell with what any doctor says, I can heal myself.

This worked for a while. Like I said, it was a good place to grab hold of some much needed self-empowerment. But such a simplistic, black-and-white way of looking at life's experience goes only so far before it collapses in upon itself. After a few months at the Healing Circle, I began to see how people used these very same beliefs and principles to drown themselves in guilt when their bodies did not "outwardly manifest" the desired healing. So-called spiritual counselors, whom I knew and had once respected, were telling friends of mine who were not getting physically better that the growing illness was their own fault; they obviously weren't thinking pure and positive enough thoughts. More than a few people came to me in shame and disgrace, thinking themselves to be failures as their diseases progressed. What had once been a momentous point of empowerment in my life had become a shaming, pointing finger, as self-righteous as any I'd ever experienced.

I remember one striking experience that occurred when I was a chaplain at Parkland. The chaplain on duty in the emergency room paged me and when I returned her call, she asked, "Could you please come down here? I've got a patient who wants me to do something called an 'Inner Guide' visualization and I don't have the slightest idea what she means. I thought you would know." (Such was my reputation at the hospital.) When I arrived at the E.R., I found a New Ager in tears. She'd been admitted for colon cancer. The doctors at the hospital out-patient cancer clinic had found that her tumor was not responding to chemotherapy. Instead, it was growing rapidly. They'd decided she needed surgery as soon as possible and sent her to the E.R. for emergency admittance into the hospital. She had come to the clinic for a routine checkup on her healing progress and ended up being prepped for the operating table instead. Understandably, she was emotionally wrecked. But—and here's the most amazing thing—

she wasn't distraught because of the cancer itself and its implications (that fear would come later, of course). She was devastated because she had "failed" at thinking positively enough.

She begged me for help in reaching her Inner Guide since she didn't know what to do and had nowhere else to turn. After directing her along a basic Inner Guide visualization (and not really to her satisfaction either—no direct magical answer to her dilemma was forthcoming), I did a bit of probing. "Do you belong to any support group?" I asked. She told me she did, but then confessed she couldn't count on anyone from her group showing up at the hospital. "It's a positive-thinking group. And I'm such a failure at trying to think positive thoughts. They'll all know that now, for sure. None of them will ever come here. To come to the hospital is to let in negative energy, you know."

This form of spiritual guilt is more commonplace than might be suspected, and it's certainly not limited to New Age spirituality. It is quite prevalent in many fundamentalist Christian circles and also found in some Eastern traditions, especially in regard to taking pain medications. The basic guilt involves a misunderstanding that disease or any painful manifestation within the human body is caused by a spiritual weakness or deficiency on the sick person's behalf—as if the spiritually fit should equal the physically fit. One would think that a good look at the long list of holy men and women who have been plagued with physical pains and illnesses throughout their lives (and deaths) would rebut this shaky theory, but amazingly this is not so. It seems to defy common sense. Clearly, another look is in order. In his book on the power of prayer in medicine, *Healing Words*, physician Larry Dossey addresses this issue directly:

> Plants, animals, birds, and fishes get sick, just as we do. In many instances they develop illnesses quite similar to our own, including cancer, arthritis, and bacterial and viral infections. They run headlong into accidents and trauma, and they too have the problems of old age and senility. Yet when animals or plants get sick, we take a different attitude toward them. We do not judge or blame them. We do not say that a tree is less a tree because it develops cancer or is infested with borers. It is not a dog's "fault" that it develops hip dysplasia, and a cat is not innately defective because it comes down with feline leukemia. In nature the occurrence of disease is considered a part of the natural order, not a sign of ethical, moral, or spiritual weakness. . . . We are a part of nature no less than other creatures. The kindness, forgiveness, and gentleness we extend to them when they develop disease could well be extended to ourselves.

About three months after we began the Healing Circle, one of our regular attendees died of AIDS. Many of us opened our hearts, some of us cried. But there was a definite undercurrent of "Well, if Jamie had only thought positively enough . . ." And I knew something was terribly wrong. I, and those core supporters of the group, had to take another look at what we were practicing, teaching, and believing. Our first "another look" had brought us to reject the doomsday prophecy of modern medicine and to hurriedly embrace the positive outlook of "mind over matter" metaphysics. For those of us who were willing to take yet another look (and another and another), we found that we needed to develop *a continual willingness to change*. A lot of resistance arose from the group as a whole. Many people did not want to look beyond the "love and light, all is perfect" mentality. Within several months our weekly group numbered around a dozen. But numbers were never the goal, personal growth and healing was. And we were healing. We were continually taking another look.

Our guided visualizations began to move away from outward physical healing and started emphasizing inner peace. We left behind "prosperity consciousness" for "conscious living" and, eventually, "conscious dying." Our reading list no longer included the works of pop New Age self-healing authors, but instead, conscious-dying advocates like Stephen Levine. Bit by bit, the crystals that once adorned the center of the Healing Circle were replaced by more candles, or the names of friends who had died, or various sacred objects from different spiritual traditions—someone's family Bible, a statue of the Buddha, a bird's feather. The Healing Circle was maturing, as was our definition of healing.

For me personally, what began as "I do not want to die" and then progressed to "I want to heal my body" was changing too. I was finding that the basic idea of *who I am* was expanding. I was healing something much more than my physical self. I was healing an emotional self and learning to forgive grievances held deep within the secret, protected places of my psyche. I was forgiving myself for perceived wrongdoings of childhood, forgiving my family and friends, and so growing emotionally and psychologically. In short, I was healing a love deficiency, not an immune deficiency. A relational self, an emotional self, a spiritual self—I was healing into an awareness of a "whole self" that was much more encompassing than the limited identity of my physical body.

Healing no longer meant what it used to. Then, just when I thought I had healing figured out to be some "whole life healing," I took yet another look. This was during my chaplaincy work with AIDS patients at Parkland. And this time, healing cracked wide open beyond any of my previous definitions. I began to sense that healing was a much bigger game than I'd previously thought. *Healing was about God!* My whole life was part of some inexplicable greater healing. I began to suspect that birth was a healing and—this was very radical to me at the time—so was death. With my extensive patient contact at Parkland, I experienced firsthand how a person can literally "heal into" death. A year earlier, had anyone told me that healing and dying could be the same thing, I'd have laughed aloud. In the old way of looking at death, death is healing's opposite and enemy. But as I took another look, a look from my growing and awakening perspective, death revealed itself to be an integral, even essential part of true healing.

Conscious-dying advocate Stephen Levine begins his book *Healing Into Life and Death* with a story about a cancer patient, Robin, who after years of steady focus on healing her cancer, had finally become overwhelmed by the intense pain of her disease. And so she asked, "Should I stop trying to heal and just let myself die?" He writes:

> Her question penetrated my body and froze my mind in place. I looked into her eyes, unable to respond from anything I knew or had ever experienced.
>
> Clearly it was a question only the heart could answer. And my heart, knowing deeper, whispered, "The

real question is, 'Where is healing to be found?' " It is the question life asks itself: "What is completion?" ...

As healing became more of an investigation than a preconception, Robin's pain began to diminish. The deeper she explored her process, asking, "At what level is healing to be found?", the less her original question about life as opposed to death arose. A few weeks into this process, Robin requested a healing circle. Several well-known healers came to form a circle about her and to channel into her body whatever energy might serve to heal. There was a powerful laying-on of hands. A few friends, observing from just outside the circle, said the energy was quite palpable. There was no question about the "presence of healing" in the room.

A week later Robin discovered thirty new tumors on her scalp and back, and told me, "The healing worked, my heart has never felt more open, and it seems the disease is coming to completion."

Indeed, it seemed "the healing had worked." In the weeks before she died, she spoke of experiencing a sense of wholeness she had never known.

Probably the greatest misconception we have about death and dying is that they somehow represent failure. I think we all feel this to some degree. I know I did (and still do at times—if I'm honest). It takes courage to take another look at death and not see it as failure, but instead to witness a healing process that journeys beyond the body, beyond physical life and death. That courage of taking another look is at the heart of living our dying. And it is a way of looking at death that can't be faked or adopted as merely an intellectual understanding. We have to come to feel it in our innermost beings, in our bones. We must take another look at healing and dying to see them not as opposites, but as interrelated events along an ongoing process toward greater growth and learning. It is the work of a lifetime.

Religious and Spiritual Traditions
Most religious and spiritual traditions offer guidance and counsel on how we are supposed to live our dying. But it is my experience that too often, too quickly, we take religious teachings and try to use them to avoid our real feelings and emotions. Often we embrace a religious framework in an attempt to escape our dying and, so, our living. I know I did. At one time in my journey I desperately wanted "the Answer" so I could convince myself that Everything Is Going To Be Just Fine (if not here, at least in the afterlife). With my newly adopted intellectual guideline I was then able to detour around any authentic feelings of fear, the real emotional doors through which I needed to pass.

One fact of human nature is that we usually adopt a spiritual "talk" so we don't have to feel the pain of our worldly "walk," a walk that is unavoidably headlong into pain, suffering, and eventual death. Then we can intellectualize that we don't have to really *feel* and experience and *live* our dying because we're in Jesus' merciful hands; or because Buddha taught reincarnation and we've got plenty of lives to live again; or because bodily death is an illusion; or because we're no longer "attached"; or because, since we obey all the rules and keep the faith, we'll be rewarded later; or . . . whatever. We've all experienced this spiritual bypass in action. It goes nowhere. Ultimately, we end up back where we started, having to face the very fears and pain we so desperately wished to avoid in the first place. Though some religions (misguidedly, I think) encourage these "blind faith" bypasses, I believe that the authentic source from which our great religions sprang, encouraged just the opposite. At their authentic foundations, I believe the great religions invite us to live our dying and consciously explore the impermanence of our human life experience.

Questioning our religious assumptions is integral to living our dying. Those who are not ready to take another look will discourage us, saying that to question is blasphemous. They may even denounce us. Most of the great seekers and questioners have encountered this resistance from the organized religious institutions of their time: Jesus, Buddha, Saint Francis, Meister Eckhart, to name just a few. If you are ready to question, remember, you are in good company historically.

A healthy and open-minded spiritual advisor should welcome your serious questioning and refusal to accept religious doctrine blindly. All true teachers cherish a sincerely questioning student. They recognize your sincerity in searching for truth. If they don't, my advice is to find another spiritual advisor or teacher. Find a support system that works for you, one that allows you to grow and question *in the light of dying*. Also, you can have more than one teacher, and your teachers need not be limited to living people, either. Read books, rent videotapes, listen to what the checkout person at the local market tells you. Each is your teacher. Don't limit yourself.

I remember how startled I was when one of my teachers told me, "If you can't find a religion that supports you, start your own." Then she pointed out that every religion was started by someone, somewhere who was dissatisfied with what the existing religions at the time had to offer. At first this seemed somewhat blasphemous, but I've since come to understand that we must each take responsibility for our own personal spiritual path. Consider this: it is your experience of the sacred and yours alone that you are embarked upon. As the Catholic monk Thomas Merton wrote:

> First of all, although men have a common destiny, each individual also has to work out his own personal salvation for himself. . . . We can help one another to find the meaning of life no doubt. But in the last analysis, the individual person is responsible for living his own life and for "finding himself." If he persists in shifting his responsibility to somebody else, he fails to find out the meaning of his own existence. You cannot tell me who I am, and I cannot tell you who you are. If you do not know your own identity, who is going to identify you?

Do not be afraid to question what scriptures or spiritual teachers tell you in the light of your own personal experience with death and dying. Your experience is here, in part, to challenge you to do just that exploration. If the teaching reflects truth, your experience with dying will strengthen your former belief into experiential knowing. It is the experiential knowing that heals and awakens, not the belief itself.

Suffering, Pain, and Spiritual Practices

There is a misunderstanding amongst some spiritual seekers that exploring the finite limitations of our human nature will threaten the infinite spiritual reality of our limitless soul's nature. This is akin to saying the way to heaven is through denying and ignoring our worldly pain and suffering. It is a popular misunderstanding and polarization: human emotional pain versus holy perfection. Another look is called for in regard to spirit and pain. Let's consider the Christian tradition first.

Certainly Jesus himself demonstrated again and again that he was very present to those who suffered around him. He did not and, I believe, *could not* deny the pain and torment of his earthly life experience. Upon hearing of Lazarus' death, he wept like any other human. He was quick to defend the oppressed and downtrodden, even at the risk of his own life. He felt the agonizing pain of betrayal when his closest friends rejected his teaching and didn't live up to his expectations. More than once he lost his compassion and equanimity in a raging fit, cursing and condemning whole populations to burn in hell. He was, in many respects, as human as you or I. Yet one of his holy qualities that most of us have not yet mastered was his ability to embrace both the so-called light and dark sides of humankind. He befriended tax collectors, the crooked law enforcement officers for Rome; one of his best friends and constant companions was Mary Magdalen, a prostitute; he hung out with lepers (the AIDS patients of his time); the list of socially unacceptable people he befriended is extensive. He looked into our hearts and saw no distinctions. To him, human beings were children of God who each had a limitless soul existing beyond birth or death. It was toward this limitless nature in us that Jesus resonated. He saw us for who we truly are—an act that was exemplified when he forgave the very people who crucified him, understanding that "they know not what they do." My aim in all this is not to give a lesson in biblical interpretation, but simply to point out that Jesus certainly *felt* his human emotions and *embraced* the worldly reality of what appears as life's darker side—which includes pain, suffering, and dying.

As I read the great spiritual teachings of the world, they each ask us to befriend and embrace our own pain and suffering as a key to the Way. Buddhism may be a bit more direct in this with its overt emphasis on life's impermanence. As an American Zen master bluntly says, " 'I certainly am going to die.' It's something we could meditate on, keeping in front of us all the time." The message seems to be: it is within *this* worldly life's built-in obsolescence that we find our way to another life—a life beyond our birth and death, of wholeness and indivisibility with God and all things. This is the sacred paradox. So many of us want to jump into that Eternal Life without first embracing the very mortal and suffering-filled Way to it. Yet, it is as St. Francis of Assisi prayed, it is in our dying that we are born back into the eternal life of God's wholeness.

Our spiritual practices will not save us from pain and confusion. Instead, they show us that avoidance of pain does not really help. It is only in being fully alive and present to the situation, in honoring whatever *is*, that we move further. False spirituality may provide "the Answer" as a defense against life's uncertainties and suffering—"an inoculation," as Joseph Campbell called popular religion, to avoid the unknown. But true spirituality leads into that very same unknown, into the whole mysterious process of living and dying. True spirituality is a continual movement away from the certainty of "This is the Answer" and toward a larger, more inclusive attitude of questioning. How easily our spiritual practices are distorted in order to bring us comfort, instead of growth. We become confused, thinking our spirituality is here to inoculate us against experiencing pain and our fears of death.

In his book *A Path With Heart*, Jack Kornfield shares excerpts from a letter written by a man hospitalized for a heart attack:

> Never have I known the experiences and sufferings which attended my stay in Intensive Care. Due to powerful medicines, unending injections, and oxygen tubes just to breathe, my mind was overcome with pain and confusion. I realized that it is extremely difficult to maintain awareness without becoming confused during the stages of death. At its worst, forty-one days after I became ill, the condition of my body was such that I became the lord of a cemetery, my mind was like that of an anti-God and my speech like the barking of an old mad dog.

The man who wrote this letter is Tibetan meditation master Lama Yeshe, considered to be one of the most compassionate and enlightened teachers of our century. As he shows us, no matter how spiritually advanced, we cannot avoid troubles with sickness and death. And to lose our balance and grounding in the midst of pain is natural. That loss is part of the process too. We are used to living in our heads, especially in matters regarding spirituality. Why not try living in our bodies for a while? Why not be real about what we're experiencing?

Lama Yeshe's experience did not stop with his deep detour into fear and hopelessness. As he continued to awaken to his own dying process, he was eventually able to move through his confusion and into peace. Though his spiritual practices did not save him from experiencing pain and confusion, they did help him facilitate the process of *movement through* those experiences.

When we take another look at our spiritual practices we begin to see that their purpose is not to inoculate us from pain, but to provide us with tools with which to process and transform seemingly meaningless pain into meaningful growth experiences. When we begin to suspect a greater meaning to our experience, we begin to learn life's lessons without self-judgment and criticism. We begin to prepare the fertile soil for our own growth in sacred self-awareness.

God

And just what about God in all this? Is God, as C. S. Lewis asked, merely a "Cosmic Sadist" who in this life "hurts us beyond our worst fears and beyond all we can imagine?" Everyone asks a question like this at one time or another. How could a loving God allow all this suffering and pain? Is heaven really deaf to our cries? Where is God now, when we need Him most?

These are big questions, and not to be answered quickly or lightly. Perhaps they're not to be answered at all. Just experienced. Just lived openly and honestly. The problem with our answers is they're only words. We need experience beyond concepts and words—a knowing that passes human understanding, as the Apostle Paul said. These are questions to be honestly experienced not merely with an outsider theology, but with an inner knowing. The value of living our dying is that it continually invites us to live our daily worldly walk *prior* to our spiritual talk.

There was a riddle the chaplains used as a teaching tool/reminder when I was at Parkland Hospital. To set up the riddle, understand that Parkland's emergency room is famous (and infamous) not just because Kennedy died there, but because it is one of the busiest and best in the world. Twenty-four hours a day it is buzzing, usually overflowing with medical emergencies and critical social situations in the waiting rooms where families and friends of victims, victimizers, you name it, all walk a delicate line of fear, rage, and intolerable grief. At Parkland, an acute-care hospital with over a thousand beds, there is a chaplain whose sole assignment is working the emergency room and its waiting area. No chaplaincy work is more stressful. Our riddle went something like this:

Question: How do you tell a five-year-old child how much God loves her when her mother has just died on the E.R. operating table?

Answer: You don't.

As chaplains at Parkland it was not our job to educate people about God and His ways. We were to listen and empower, to elicit feelings and further the patient's emotional process when appropriate. And we were certainly not to truncate any movement through a natural process (such as grief, anger, fear, etc.) unless it somehow interfered with the nurses' or doctors' ability to do their job. The old-fashioned model of the chaplain is the priest on the television series M*A*S*H telling a soldier, "Don't worry, son, just have faith because you're in God's loving hands." But our process-oriented model at Parkland involved a different sort of faith and trust—a faith in a larger inexplicable process of life at work, which includes grief, anger, and dying. If a patient needed to rail at God, curse Him, question Him, deny Him, so be it. If a patient needed to seek refuge in God even to the point of extreme denial, so be it as well. Though in cases of borderline denial, I'd almost always try to elicit some honest reaction as to what a person was feeling—a forward movement in the process from denial to awareness. Ultimately, however, it was up to the individual whether or not to be honest with his or her feelings about the situation and/or about God. (And besides, while we are taking another look at it, who's to say denial is always such a bad thing? Quite often, denial is an appropriate survival response. Believe me, the last place you want to take away someone's coping mechanism—like denial— is in the middle of a high-crisis situation like Parkland's emergency room. If we're really coming to trust and have faith in a greater process of life, we need to make room for the process of denial, as well.)

As I grew in my own illness, I experienced the phenomenon of "Here's what God thinks about you and your illness" from the other side, the ill person's side. I can't tell you how much spiritual shaming is done in the guise of offering encouraging words and spiritual advice about God and His ways. And it can be extremely subtle. Yesterday, an old friend from my earlier "self-healing" days called. I'd not spoken to him in over four years. Of course he asked, "How are you feeling?" It has become a practice of mine to be very honest with this question—even though most people don't really want to hear the truth. I take this obligation as part of my "living our dying" activism. (And I do consider living our dying an activist stance in this culture.) So I told him, "Actually, I'm feeling much better now than I have been in the last year or so. My neuropathy is not so severe and I'm feeling more energy. But you know, since you last saw me, my body has changed. Outwardly, I look healthy enough. But I probably have a quarter of the stamina and energy I did when you knew me. I'm fatigued a lot of the time."

There was a long silence. Then I caved in. "But, I'm fine overall, really."

A sigh of relief from my old friend. That's what he wanted to hear. I'd been his spiritual advisor and role model. There was a belief that I would never get sick or die. ("Because as long as Joseph lives, there's hope for me.") Remember, in our old model it was spiritually incorrect to admit our disease's progression and physical vulnerability— the underlying rule being that the "spiritual" way to proceed was to always focus on the positive. It's often no less true today. Usually when I am asked about my latest work and I reply, "A book titled *Living Our Dying*," I receive an awkward silence in response. To mention dying and death is still mostly taboo. Sometimes people counter with something like, "But you aren't really dying, are you? You don't think that?" And occasionally someone even says something akin to, "Have you given up hope *that* much?" Most of us still believe dying to be an extremely taboo, not to mention ungodly, topic to speak about. This is the importance of the basic practices outlined in Chapter 2: they begin to undo that taboo quality and awkwardness we associate with bringing death and dying out of their closet.

I believe a great deal of the spiritual bypassing done on God's behalf—such as avoiding the topic of death, or dismissing it quickly with "She's in God's loving hands now"—has something to do with a deep suspicion of God. We don't want to come to that door marked "Anger at God" and push through it. (This is partially because we're afraid we might discover that God is indeed a cruel sadist, as C. S. Lewis wondered, or—even worse—that God doesn't really care one way or the other.) But the true seeker will not allow that door to rest unopened. Our awakening depends on opening and facing those hidden fears. We must go deeper.

You will have to come to your own understanding about God and the fact that you and others are dying. The key here is the future tense, "will have to come." Though you may have read various understandings that resonate within you—and, so, in a way you do understand somewhat because you have a belief in place—remember, you understand only from your perspective now. And, believe me, that perspective is often growing, changing. I know of nothing that facilitates this movement more than the daily effort and practice of living our dying. This is part of the journey into sacredness. In this world we're trained to fear the ever-changing and unknown, but as we take another look, we can see their holiness. The point is certainly not that you agree with my personal understanding of God but that *you come to your own understanding in light of the continual growth and re-evaluation that dying affords*. Leave no sacred cows outside of this re-evaluation. This earthly time in life is your opportunity to look at them all.

"Jesus Saves"

When I first visited Tim, he was on a respirator and expected to live only a couple of days. His brother and sister-in-law had recently arrived from Kentucky with the news that his mother couldn't come. Tim was disappointed at first, but was so happy to see his brother that it seemed to make up for the loss. The disease, or the medication, had blurred his thinking process to the extent that Tim was sure he was going to be released from the hospital in order to return home to Kentucky within the next few days. He kept telling everyone that his mother was coming to Dallas to take him home to Kentucky with her, that she loved him so much she was coming herself. When his brother found out I was the chaplain, he asked to see me privately.

At the time, there was no counseling room available, so we ended up alongside the busy and crowded corridor of Parkland's ninth-floor east wing. The rush of people passing by provided its own privacy. For some awkward moments the young man just stood there, looking at his large hands that were held together in front of him like he was wearing handcuffs. He just stared down at those hands.

The brother was a big bear of a man in his mid-twenties. He was from a rural town, wore jeans and a blue work shirt, the kind with his name stitched above the pocket, like a mechanic. I asked him the chaplain's number-one question: "What's this experience like for you?" And he looked up, directly into my eyes.

"My momma ain't gonna come. She hopes Tim

hurries up and dies. She's had to lie to everyone about what he's got. If the other people in our church found out, it'd just about kill our momma." I noticed his baseball cap. It said "Jesus Saves" across the front.

I just repeated softly, "How does all this make *you* feel?"

"I don't want Tim to go to hell." He was looking down at his cuffed hands again. "But I know he's gonna. He's sinned and now he's payin' for it. You understand that, bein' a pastor. Our pastor back home explained it all to us before we came."

My job, as I saw it, was not to give theological instruction unless asked, but rather to share the experience of love directly and surely by my presence. So, what could I say? What could I say that would be *of love* through me, and not of my theological beliefs—which were not exactly in accord with those of Tim's brother?

He continued. "What am I gonna do about Tim? The doctors say he'll die in a couple of days. But what am I gonna do? He's a sinner. What do I say to him?"

What do I say to him? That was my question too. What do I say here? The bustling noise of the corridor kept us isolated in our seeking. What, just what? The brother waited.

Carefully, I took the man by both his hands to get his complete attention. "What do you think Jesus would say to Tim, if he were here now?"

Tim's brother said nothing and all of Parkland seemed to pause in silence with him. A few seconds later he nodded his head simply, as if understanding. He looked me directly in my eyes. He said, "Jesus would forgive him. And tell Tim that he loves him."

Once again, in the words of C. S. Lewis, "My idea of God is not a divine idea. It has to be shattered time after time. He shatters it Himself. He is the great iconoclast. Could we not almost say that this shattering is one of the marks of His presence?"

A warning about the journey: inevitably, as I write about this process, it will appear as if living our dying follows some linear progression from A to B to C. It is so tempting to think, "Ah, now I am at C and when I progress further along I will be at D, never having to revisit C again." But this formulaic, linear line of thinking is a misunderstanding. The fact is, wherever we are in our process, we are constantly taking another look. So please don't think that after we do our "practices" in Chapter 2, we "take another look" at life in Chapter 3, and then go on to Chapter 4, never having to "take another look" or do our "practices" again. The journey is not so nicely linear. We don't begin at A and progress one letter at a time to Z. Life is more like alphabet soup than the alphabet song.

Taking another look at our world is an ongoing act. It's not an answer in itself, just a movement along the journey.

The Self That Doesn't Die

When I was five years old, we moved into a new neighborhood. One of my favorite places was the large field behind our lot. It was bigger than a football field. My first friends in the neighborhood were three baby toads and a praying mantis who lived in the field. Playing back there, I could lose my loneliness as the new kid on the block.

It wasn't long before I met the human inhabitants of the neighborhood. George, a year younger than me, lived in the house next to ours. George introduced me to Corgi toy cars and make-believe races along his driveway. I introduced him to the field and the toads and mantis. Quickly the secret field began to transform. With two fertile imaginations, our field became a war zone for cops and robbers, cowboys, and Indians. As the other kids from the neighborhood joined us, an oasis of nature was gentrified. We played that summer as if the world were coming to an end. And in a way it was—first grade was about to begin. Real school, not kindergarten.

Late one fall day after school, George and I were playing G.I. Joe in the field, when George dropped his plastic machine gun and just started off, up to the horizon, toward the trees. The tall oaks that had once cushioned us with their thick green leaves, separating the field into its own private galaxy, were now baring naked branches. In the distance was a neighborhood we had never seen before. George pointed to the rooftop of a house in the distance.

"Mamaw lives there," he blurted. We both just stared in silence for a while.

I was as stunned as George by the sudden realization. The idea of someone's grandma—delectable, hugging, engulfing, gift-giving creatures that all grandmas were— the idea of one of those living so close! (Mine were over an hour drive away by car, in Mineola, Texas.) A grandma so close, so accessible. This meant I could go there myself without my parents driving me. I'd assumed it was a universal law that all grandmas lived at least an hour away.

Over the next several weeks, at my insistence, we finally visited George's Mamaw. And it was true. She was every bit as delicious as my own. (Ice-cold milk and crisp crumbly Oreo cookies every visit.) For that first visit, George's mom drove us in her new Cadillac. It wasn't too long, however, before George and I crossed our shrinking galaxy of a field for ourselves to arrive at Mamaw's house independently, under our own power. Throughout the rest of the school year, George and I made several journeys to Mamaw's for milk and Oreo cookies.

In early summer, Mamaw died. I remember my

mother sitting on my bed, patting her hand softly to the spot beside her. "Joe, honey, I've got something to tell you." By the hollow, unsure tone of her voice, I knew that something bad had happened. When I sat beside her, she told me. "George's Mamaw has gone to heaven and is with God now." My mother seemed so stiff. I nodded as though I understood what she was saying to me. And in a way, I did.

George and I never talked about his Mamaw after that. Somehow we knew we weren't supposed to. Just like the grown-ups didn't talk about her. It was my first encounter with human death.

I remember the following fall, when the tall oaks once again parted themselves and I saw the rooftop of what had once been Mamaw's house. As usual, George and I were playing make-believe in the field. Everything was there: the sky, the sun, the mockingbirds and praying mantis, a new batch of baby toads, and George beside me. Mamaw was in that field too. I felt her there. But I said nothing about it. I didn't think the grown-ups would understand.

It has been said that ever since *Genesis* pointed out that God created man in His own image, the aim of theological studies became "know thyself." For those of us serious about our spiritual process, this understanding of aim or purpose helps. But in our hearts we know that the journey is much more than simply coming to understand the human self, or ego. Of course a healthy understanding of ego-self functioning is important—we call it psychology—but such an understanding could not be the totality of the journey's purpose. There has to be more.

To truly heal, the journey of awakening must transcend beyond the human ego-based self into another more sacred "self." To truly heal, we must each come to that holy self *Genesis* speaks of—that self originally created in God's own image. The return to this sacred, eternal self-awareness is the journey's purpose.

Though the names given it differ, every religion I'm aware of speaks of this eternal self that is never born and never dies. In Christianity we think of this self as our soul nature, which once fully developed, is known as "Christ consciousness." (In the *New Testament*, the Apostle Paul calls this inner potential the "mind of Christ;" and in the Catholic tradition, it is exemplified by sainthood.) Hindus know this eternal self as the "Atman." For Buddhists, it is the enlightened recognition of "Buddha nature."

Often disciples and students confuse the teacher's personality and ego-self with the eternal self. This basic confusion can be found in every spiritual tradition. Yet each self-awakened teacher I'm aware of taught that this potential to realize self is universal—that within each person there is the seed, the potential, to awaken to holy self. For example, as a human being on a spiritual journey, Jesus realized that he and "the Father" were one identity. At times he made the distinction that Jesus-the-man was merely the external instrument—"It is not I but the Father that dwells within me who does the work." At other times he spoke from his realized Christed identity—"I and the Father are one." Central to his teaching throughout, however, was the fact that "the kingdom of God is within you" too.

Likewise, Buddhist teachings tell us that we are each potential Buddhas; Buddha nature lives within us all. To a Buddhist our life, here, in body is to be spent working to awaken that eternal self nature. Living in a way that is in accord with awakening the Buddha within is the practical aspect of Buddhist spiritual teachings. No less is true with the authentic Christian teachings of Jesus. As I've studied the lives and teachings of other spiritually realized persons, I've found that essentially each teacher espoused the same thing: within each of us the eternal self awaits awakening—in other words, the light is within me and you, too. Remember, it was Jesus himself who said to his followers, "greater works than I do, you shall do."

The ultimate aim of religion is to help us regain our lost awareness of this inner sacred self—to continue the human race's awakening into sacred self, to do "greater works" as Jesus said. The true religious question is about finding the way toward this remembrance or realization of self. It is a question of "how." How do we come to live in the awareness of this eternal self, while living here in this temporal world and body? How do we reflect, through our human lives, now, this eternal knowledge of God's Reality? How do we grow in that eternal awareness daily?

Our world's spiritual traditions each offer methods and practices whose aim is sacred self-awakening. For example, in Buddhism there is sitting and walking meditation; in Taoism, tai chi; in Christianity, worship, fasting, a life of sacrifice and service, contemplative prayer. Hinduism, Catholicism, Protestantism, Methodism, Judaism, Native American spirituality, all have specific methods and practices aimed at directing the seeker closer toward experiencing the sacred. Bringing a conscious awareness to living our dying is not meant to replace any of these practices. Awakening to dying will, however, enrich the environment and intention in which our other spiritual practices are performed. It is commonplace nowadays to hear spiritual teachers speaking of cancer, AIDS, and other life-threatening illness as "the accelerated course" in spiritual awakening. Consciously living our dying is one of the most powerful ways to assist us in the inner work of cultivating sacred self-awareness.

As we honestly come up against our own edges of fear and denial about the "little I" that is born, grows old, and dies in time, we will also come to recognize another "I am" that is eternal.

Planes of Consciousness

Conscious-dying advocate Ram Dass, whose spiritual training is basically from Eastern traditions, offers a metaphor for understanding the vastness of sacred self that we in the West can easily grasp: the different channels we see on television. He asks us to consider that we see and experience our reality through a little television that is placed in front of our eyes. Imagine all we can see is that television's picture. It completely fills our view. The various channels available on our television correspond to the various "planes of consciousness" or "levels of reality" we allow ourselves to perceive. For example, most people in our Western culture believe we have only one or two channels available to us, whereas the truth, Ram Dass says, is that we have many available. Instead of a one- or two-channel limitation, we have cable; most of us just aren't aware of it yet. The metaphor extends like this:

We begin by identifying the first basic channel we all receive. It views our personal reality in terms of physical bodies. It sees old, young, light, dark, fat, thin, all the physical traits and appearances of other bodies. As newborn human beings, this is the first channel we learn to watch. And though its limitations become quickly obvious with experience, it still remains our original channel, the most accessible and comfortable.

The second channel is far more interesting. In this realm we see type-A-achiever lawyers, neurotic artists, unfulfilled housewives, enthusiastic spiritual seekers, and shy librarians. This channel views our personal realities through the psycho-social domain. From here we categorize our world and people in terms of psychological attributes: happy, sad, wounded, depressed, manic, and so forth. We also see in terms of social roles, such as banker, housewife, college professor, blue- or white-collar worker. Add to that Republican, Democrat, Marxist, atheist, communist, Episcopalian, the list goes on. This is a fascinating, almost endless channel to play around within. Most people in our culture see life primarily through these first two channels. Ask someone, "Who are you?" and listen to the response. It is almost always limited to either channel 1 or 2.

What happens if we flick to the next channel on our television? To the surprise of many, there are other channels.

In the next channel—one that is still very low in the ratings but that has gained some new audience of late—we find what might be described as the "astral plane" of consciousness. This is the plane where Jungian archetypes are seen, the realm of mythic identities. From here we see people not in their physical, psychological, or social roles, but in their mythological structures. Certain schools of contemporary psychological thought, particularly those based on the teachings of Carl Jung, are making great headway into this channel. Therapist-authors such as James Hillman (*Re-Visioning Psychology*) and Thomas Moore (*Care of the Soul* and *Soul Mates*) have come a long way in opening our eyes to this channel's existence. From here we look out at other people and see the myth of Narcissus, the self-absorbed youth, or Odysseus, the longing father, being re-enacted upon our individual as well as collective psyche-astral planes. (By the way, astrology and tarot cards may also be considered more popular forms of this channel.)

If we switch the channel again, we come to a plane of consciousness that exists behind all the individual and mythological differences. From this channel we look out at other people and do not see differences, we see sames. From here we see other souls on a spiritual journey just like us. We are not merely human beings having a spiritual experience, but spiritual beings having merely a human experience. Brief, fleeting moments of access to this channel are more common than widely reported. It happens most often with infants and young children. We're talking baby-talk to a child and for a moment, something shifts, and we become suddenly aware that there's another soul in there, in that little body, looking out at us. For a split second we're not older, mature adults holding a child, we're fellow travelers on a journey. Sometimes we are even aware that the child's soul may seem much older or more developed than our own. We feel the presence of a wise yet timeless being. In the everyday world, this switch to the "Fellow Soul-Traveler Channel" happens far less often between two adults. Usually it is only after we begin consciously embracing a spiritual path that we occasionally begin to watch the world through this channel again.

This is an important channel for us to recognize when we're working on living our dying. From here we can see all the channels before—the physical body that has cancer or AIDS, the young artist in the prime of his career, or the matronly grandmother in her golden years—as part of a costume or packaging that serves a soul's greater journey. From here we can begin to develop experientially a perception that sees beyond the earthly costume of form and appearance. This is where we begin to connect with the sacred self that lives beneath the personality or ego self. It is from this channel's perspective that the romantic poet William Blake could say, "I cannot think of death as more than the going out of one room into another." But it is important to understand that this channel is not to be used to deny or escape the pain we experience through earlier channels; far from it. Rather, by experientially recognizing this level of reality, we can come to move more gracefully through and transform the pain we experience in earlier channels. By spending time in this channel, we can begin to cultivate the courage, understanding, and compassion to be wholly present and alive to our earlier self identities because, in light of this channel's truth, we are not so easily swept away into the fears and extra baggage we carry regarding our bodily (channels 1 and 2) death.

Consider it this way: when an infant screams out

in pain because of baby teeth coming in, of course we still empathize with her predicament; in a figurative manner, we feel her pain with her. Yet, as adults who see a bigger picture, we aren't swept away into screaming agony as is the infant. In the very face of what is so overwhelming to the infant, part of us might even be aware of feeling a joy and appreciation for the wonder of life's greater unfolding. Spending time in the Fellow Soul-Traveler Channel allows us to develop a broader perspective toward death and dying. However, as with all parts of the journey, it is one thing to intellectually understand that this channel exists, and quite another to actually view life through it.

So far, it has been relatively easy to comprehend the different channels of perceptual reality. The next channel is not so conceptually familiar. This is the channel where our fellow soul-travelers disappear and we are left seeing only "the One." This is the channel the mystic sees in her raptures. From here, we are all the Ancient One. Even though we recognize that the One has become the many— the myriad of forms in the world, the others—we see behind the many and into our One Shared Self. When we look at another person, we don't see another body, personality, or soul-traveler, we see the "One That Is Who I Am." It's as if a giant mirror were held up before us everywhere we look. From here, there is just One looking at itself. This is not metaphorical or intellectual; it is real. All the previous channels are now understood to be only relatively real, symbolic separations in order to play (or as the Hindus say, dance) out the drama of life. But is this channel "more real" than the previous? This we cannot say. Every reality up to this point is an equally valid experiential reality. From the perspective of the One, we cannot separate our previous realities as unreal; from here, it is All Real. (In other words, we only make these distinctions of separate planes or levels from a pre-One perspective. To the One, such distinctions are meaningless.) As pointed out, this is a highly mystical plane of consciousness. Obviously we cannot exist solely here for too long a period of time and still function within the everyday world. This is a channel we touch upon again and again, but it is not a place we reside in for too long and still remain in body.

And there is yet another channel. One final flick of the remote switch. From here, everything disappears. All the previous channels, the subject-object distinction, the One, even the television itself disappears. All returns to the void from which all things arose. All returns to the formless that lies behind the One. In Christian, Judaic, and Muslim traditions it is God—not the God of our concepts, but God the Ineffable. For Buddhists it is Nirvana; for Hindus it is Brahma; and in Taoism it is called the Eternal Tao, the "Truth that cannot be told of"—or thought of, or conceived. The Hebrews spell this ineffable God "G-d" to emphasize that it cannot be spoken or represented, only pointed toward. And according to early Christian texts, this ineffable God remains hidden in a "cloud of unknowing" as far as the human mind's ability to understand It is concerned. This is the unspeakable, inconceivable source of all.

It is important to remember that each of us is receiving ongoing information from all these channels. It is not merely a special few who can receive them. This is the message with which we began this chapter by quoting the great teachers and founders of the world's religions, who each said the light is in you and me too. We all have the potential to receive the higher channels on our inner television. How else are we going to do greater works? Our problem, culturally and individually, is that we have defined channels 1 and 2 as the only "relevant" realities. It's not that the other channels don't exist, it's that we don't bother to switch the dial. And when we do switch the dial, or life's circumstance forces us to scan the other channels for a while, we usually receive only static. This isn't because the higher channels are not being broadcast. It is because we've so devalued the higher channels, and so busied and focused ourselves on channels 1 and 2, we just can't see anything else without retraining and undoing our previous assumptions—without radically taking another look. Remember, according to a world that values only channels 1 and 2, the higher channels are always classified as an "error" in reception. This book began by asking you to consider those times in your life when someone important to you had died and you were temporarily cast into an altered state, feeling a different texture of life and asking the bigger questions. From the perspective of channels 1 and 2, you cannot "come back to the real world" or "get back into the stream of life" fast enough. Also, consider that a mystical experience of the Oneness of all things—definitely seeing from a higher channel—is quickly diagnosed by channel 2 as a psychotic fragmentation of personal boundaries.

It also seems that the higher we go up the channels, the more upside down the lower channels appear, the more "neurotic" our channel-1 and channel-2 self appears. Telecast, so to speak, from channel 3, Jungian psychotherapy advocates embracing our former neurosis (as defined by channel 2) into a larger, mythic view of life's overall process. The higher the channel, the more potentially inclusive the view becomes (including reception of the lower channels as well).

The television-channel metaphor has been introduced in hopes of clarifying a predicament all of us encounter when we begin to work on living our dying. The predicament is that, as long as we see *only* through channels 1 and 2, we will continue to be rightfully afraid of death and dying. In my experience in working with those who are nearing death, their fear comes not only from what might happen in some hellish afterlife, but in an underlying assumption that they exist only on the first two channels. To someone who has experienced reality as limited to these two channels—the physical and psychological—bodily death is obviously terrifying. It is self-extinction, the ultimate meaningless act.

Coming to experience life, to see ourselves, others, and our world, through these higher planes of reality allows us to see death from a much broader perspective. From the "Fellow Soul-Traveler" plane we look into the eyes (the mirror to the soul) of someone who's dying, and we see a fellow soul. We feel a connection that says, "Hey, are you in there? Yea, I'm out here. What an amazing journey this is, eh?" From here we can go even deeper into the present moment to communicate and heal on a soul-level. From this perspective we are allowed to experience a death on channels 1 and 2, not as the final end, but as merely a change in the outer appearance of the soul's greater process.

And, as mentioned above, perhaps one of the greatest benefits of expanding our reception of channels is that receiving higher channels allows us to experience more fully the lower (because, in light of the higher channels, we're not so swept away by our lower-channel fears). This can bring us to experience a great paradox of the soul's journey: in the lower channels there is a vast melodrama of tremendous suffering, pain, and unfairness, and we are the actors in it; but from the higher channels, we can look at channels 1, 2, and 3, at the individual dramas and differences, and honestly say, "I see the perfection of it all; I see the grace and unfolding of my soul's curriculum here."

One of the pitfalls along the spiritual journey is when the seeker mistakenly believes that the goal of the journey is to exist only on the higher planes of consciousness. There is the yearning in each of us that wants to bypass all this earthly toil and just hang out in bliss and ecstasy, looking out primarily from the "big picture." But this is not the true inner way. If we take this route, what we might call "spiritual denial," we may end up telling others or ourselves, "It's all right, don't worry; you're not a body, but a soul. This earthly pain isn't real anyway." Ask yourself, is this truly seeing the big picture, is this the compassionate and healing voice of Christed self or Buddha nature? Being attached to seeing only through the higher channels is no more liberated than being caught only in the lower: seeing only the pain, suffering, and hell of life without a meaningful context of the soul's greater journey. The true way is not to try to escape life's pain by hiding out in the higher channels (besides, it doesn't work), but to be open to it all.

We can see this yearning to hide out clearly when we work with others who are dying. How quickly we want to leap to the Fellow Soul-Traveler plane and bypass all our hidden fears and feelings about death. How quickly we want to say, "John made his transition last night," instead of, "John died." The way of living our dying cultivates a balance of living through the lower and higher channels, simultaneously. So, yes, there is room made for saying, "John dropped his body" without it necessarily indicating spiritual denial. But these are delicate, subtle distinctions and only you can truly know for yourself. Much of the remainder of this book is devoted to a deeper examination and inquiry into these subtle distinctions. Again, it is my prayer that this helps.

Who Am I?

The history of religious seeking is filled with our misunderstandings about the levels of reality and what might be defined as the sacred self. For some this self has become a goal, something placed "outside" of us, something to achieve and possess; for others it has been idealized as the "good," whereas the human personality or ego has been branded "evil." In reality, the sacred self cannot be so easily grasped or defined. Conceptually, we are unequipped to wholly understand it. Self is not another one of the objects of our world to be studied, analyzed, and codified. Self is the quintessential subject itself. The holy self of God, which is within us all, exists as the Original Subject long before our conceptual thinking apparatus entered consciousness. Instead of speaking of the self as a fixed thing, an object-noun, we can better understand it as a fluid relationship of movements and experience. The eternal self is a verb, an ongoing unfolding of God's experience now, in this very life—"the existing" in all planes of consciousness simultaneously. And the paradox is, "You are That."

The true religious question asks, How can we begin to make room for the appearance of self in our daily life? The beloved Indian Saint Ramana Maharshi taught his students that an inquiry in the form of "Who am I?" was the principal means to the realization of self. Of course, by this Sri Ramana didn't mean that we need only walk around asking, "Who am I, who am I?" all day long. He was speaking of a more sincere endeavor, a vital inquiry in which nothing else is more important.

The spiritual journey of awakening is the recognition of one's own sacred self identity. I am not a human being having a spiritual experience, but a spiritual being having a human experience. Try this: look at your hand, the one that is holding this book. Look at it closely. Now, really inquire, ask, "Is this hand *I*?"

Is this hand *I*?

Or would it be more meaningful to ask, "Is this hand *mine*?" Find the answer within. Don't jump to conclusions. Find the reasoning beneath it. "Is this hand *I*?" or "Is this hand *mine*?"

There is a difference.

It is the difference between "I am a body" and "I am not a body, but I have one." It is a difference of identity. Who am *I*? What am *I*? What is this *I* that has a body, but is not the body? By doing this kind of exercise we can each come to the realization that this hand is not the *I*, but is *mine.* In other words, "Though I may possess my hand, I am not to be found *in* my hand."

You may try this with other parts of your body. Remember, it does little good simply to agree with what someone else says about it. The key is to find out personally. It's quite profound to discover that all this time, all this life experience, "I've been wrong about thinking that this body is *I.*"

Find out for yourself.

A Guided Meditation and Inquiry into
the Self That Doesn't Die

The following guided meditation involves the visualization of your own body's death. It follows the body's death through different dying scenarios, including a scenario emphasizing your specific life-challenging condition (if you don't have a diagnosis, imagine a dying scenario that is possible). This meditation is an inquiry into *what* you are beyond the costume of your body/personality—beyond the lower channels, and even beyond the soul-traveler plane. Remember, this is an exploration. Let go into the journey. Trust where this goes.

Prepare a quiet place for yourself where you won't be interrupted. You may try playing some gentle, instrumental music in the background as you read this. You are participating in something holy. Give yourself that space. Honor your process. Light a candle if you wish. Also, try to clear your mind with meditation or prayer before you begin. It is best to have someone you trust read this aloud to you, but it is not necessary. Or you may tape-record this in your own voice. Travel through this meditation several times.

Know that you are healing. Also, don't mistake this meditation as some cure-all spiritual method. It isn't. It is merely a tool that, like all spiritual tools, has a built-in obsolescence.

Some of us will take to this practice of guided meditations more easily than others. In doing this kind of work with large groups, I've found that usually at least one person says that "nothing happened." Don't worry. For some of us, especially those who are not so visually minded, this practice takes practice. But I've never met anyone who couldn't eventually do it. (As a teacher once said to me, "If you can describe what your bathroom at home looks like, you can visualize.") So be gentle with yourself. Try not to delve into self-attack and judgment for "not getting it." On some level the meditation will do its work. And, gradually or dramatically, you will come to experience the process this meditation invokes.

If you've done guided meditations before and are an old pro, you already understand that each time you do one, it is different. Sometimes the experience can be a breakthrough process, while at other times, it gently softens and wears away our preconceptions. I think this meditation can be a little of both. When I've done this at workshops, often it is dramatic, much of the room bursting forth with a giant experiential "ah-ha!" And just as often it has been quiet and somber (and I've wondered, "Did I say it wrong?"). Through experience I've come to understand that it is not the meditation nor my leading it that was different; it was the moment, the group's needs, my needs, God's needs. Finally, we just have to trust that we're doing our inner work and don't always understand why things are the way they are.

Though there is an end to the visualization, it actually opens into an experiential questioning. The aim is not an intellectual "I understand," but rather an experiential "ah-ha." What you are about to read may bring up some feelings of fear. If fearful thoughts and feelings arise, just pause for a moment, take a deep breath—then come back. Deep within we each recognize the truth when we hear it.

And, again, if possible, take some time to still yourself and prepare before you do this . . .

"WHO AM I, REALLY?"

[To be read slowly to a friend,
silently to yourself, or tape recorded
in your own voice.]

Sit in a comfortable position. Don't lie down. Sit up. Let yourself come to a soft, quiet place deep within you.

Let the possibilities open.

Opening . . .

Take a slow and easy deep breath.

[—inhale—]

And as you exhale, let everything go. Let go of every thought. Let go of every expectation.

Take another, even slower and deeper breath.

[—inhale—]

And this time, when you exhale, exhale with a slight sigh . . .

[—sigh—]

And relax. You are safe.

Just keep breathing. In—out. In—out. And together, we open our heart. We open the mind. We open heart and mind. Opening and opening.

No in-between. No stasis, here. No neutrality. You are either opening or closing. And we choose to open. Opening even more.

Breathing in—out. In—out.

Let your thoughts come to this very moment. This moment with you sitting, here, as you are. You are going to let your thoughts explore for a while.

Opening even more.

Now—as you sit right here, really *feel* yourself sitting. Feel what it is like to sit here, right now. Take some time with this.

[—pause for a few moments—]

In your mind's eye, *see* yourself sitting here. See yourself as though you were watching from above. As though you were watching from a nearby balcony. Looking down at yourself. Notice the expression on your face. Notice the way you carry your entire body. If there are others sitting with you, see them. See it all. Yourself sitting there with everything that's around you. Notice the whole scene down there.

Now we are going to explore. To experiment with what you see. As you watch yourself sitting, an imaginary drama will unfold. Just like a make-believe play. Just like theater. Here is our drama: it begins as a stranger comes into the scene. From your view, notice the stranger enter. And also notice that he is carrying a gun. Then, slowly, let this stranger raise the gun and point it at you. While you're sitting down there. From above, watch the drama unfold. Watch as he shoots you. Notice the smoke from the gun. The smell. The sounds. See the commotion below. Perhaps people fighting. Perhaps shock. See yourself, your body, lying on the floor. Bleeding from the gunshot wound. And let your imagination go with it.

Let your imagination fly with this scenario . . .

See the police. See the ambulance rushing through the streets.

Watching. Watching all this drama unfold. See the doctors at the hospital preparing for your arrival. See someone calling your friends and family, telling them to come to the hospital. See the pain on their faces.

Now, you are in surgery. Experience the sounds and smells of the hospital's emergency room. See and hear the beeping sounds of the heartbeat monitor. It beeps along with your pulse. See doctors and nurses working frantically over your body. The colors of the operating room. The surgical gowns. And continue to hear the heartbeat monitor. See all of this, as they work frantically over you. And then . . .

With your attention on the beeps coming from the heartbeat monitor—let the beeps stop. Let there be silence. Silence. The doctors try to resuscitate you. But whatever they try fails to work. You are dead. Silence. Watch as someone covers your body. Watch as nurses turn off the machines and life-support equipment. Watch as the drama continues after you die.

Watch as your friends and family are told that you're dead. See their pain at hearing the news. It is so painful. And then . . .

Let the scene shift quickly to your memorial service. It is now a few days later. At your memorial service. Notice where it is being held. Is it indoors or outdoors? Notice who's there. Who's not there. Notice the choice of music. Experience the whole thing. Watch it all.

And notice that "you" are still watching the drama unfold. Notice there still remains your sense of "I-am-ness." An

"I-am" who is aware of watching all this, even now. Though the body is dead, there still remains a "you" to watch these events. Look at the body, ask yourself: Is this dead body who "I-am?"

Is this dead body who I am?

[*—pause for a moment—*]

Now—bring your thoughts back to this room. Back to your present body-awareness. As you sit. Right here. Right now. Notice that you have been doing a guided meditation. Your thoughts have been "playing" with the idea that the body dies, is gone, is thought of as "you."

Take a moment and really get in touch with sitting, here. Get in touch with your feelings now, after having imagined your own death and memorial service.

And notice that you are watching yet another drama unfold. But this drama doesn't involve an imaginary gunman. This drama involves you simply sitting here. Listening to this guided meditation. But just another drama nonetheless. Watch yourself now. As you sit here. Listening.

Okay. Let's explore some more. You are going to once again imagine what it would be like to die—but this time you will die from complications arising from your own particular life-challenging condition. If it's cancer, let it be cancer. If AIDS, let it be AIDS. Leukemia, heart disease, an addiction, depression, loneliness, whatever your particular form of life-challenging condition, let it be that.

Now, let's imagine. Even more quickly this time. Picture yourself in a scenario where you are about to die from your so-called life-challenging condition. In a car perhaps. Or walking along the street. Or down a hallway. Or in a hospital bed. Wherever is most appropriate. You've thought about this before, if only for a split-second. You know this scenario of fear very well. *Go into it!* Don't wait! This time we're not going to be fearful about it—we are going to explore deeply. All is safe. This exploration is healing. *Go deep* into it.

See your body as it is, there, dying. Then see yourself die from your condition. *See the body die. Really see it.* And—even quicker—see the notification of family and friends about your death. See their reaction at hearing the news. Their faces.

And, progressing along, see the memorial service. Those gathering to remember you. Who's there? Who's not there? Let yourself experience this whole scenario, once again.

And again—notice that you are *watching* your own memorial service. You are watching the drama unfold. And notice that there still remains a "you"—an "I-am" who is watching all this, even now. The body is dead. But "I-am" still watching.

And then . . .

Let it be one year later. Your body has been dead and gone for one whole year. Notice a few of your friends or family members. Notice them one year, to the day, after your death. Notice them as they remember that "you" died a year ago. The anniversary. See them as they stop their busy lives for a moment and think of you.

Watch them, without you. Without you there in-body.

Now let your thoughts explore even more deeply. Play a game with the possibilities of life. Imagine these very same family and friends as if they had never known you. See them, there, doing whatever life has them doing, as if *you* had never been part of their lives. As if you had never been born at all.

Imagine ... Remember various times, various incidents from your life. From childhood to adulthood. Remember these incidents and see the events happening without "you" being present. All these events continue, but without "you" there. Just an empty space. See your parents. See your best friends. See those children who were mean to you as a child. See your earliest memories of school. See it all, but there is no "you" there. You are edited out. You were never born. All of it continues along just fine without "you" being there.

Now—here is our question:

If this body can die, and you can watch it happen ... If "you" could have never even been born, and you can watch that happen too ... Who are "you," really?

Think about this. Ask yourself: "Who am I? Who am I, if this body could never have been born at all?"

[—*pause*—]

It seems clear that you are *not* the body. For you can see how the body can be laid aside in many different ways. You can imagine that "death" scenario. And yet, the "I-am" still lives. You can imagine your "death" in many, many different circumstances. Yet, there is still an "I-am" that is imagining.

So, who is this "I-am" really? Who is this "I-am" that can imagine its own body's death?

"Who am *I*, really?"

[—*pause*—]

As you come deeper into this questioning, as you come into your sincerity—you may begin to understand that, at the very least, "I-am" *this awareness*.

You are *aware* of your thoughts as you think. *Aware* of sitting in a body. Of using your imaginative powers. You can be *aware* of your body dying. You can even imagine that your body never existed in the world at all. Yet still there is the *awareness*. An "I-am" that is *aware*.

Now, go even deeper. Try this. It is very simple. Try to imagine yourself *without awareness*. Really try to stop being aware of your "I-am-ness."

[—pause and really try—]

Try to have "no awareness" whatsoever . . . Really try.

[—pause and try harder—]

Ahh . . . and this is grace. Because no matter how hard you try, you will not be able to succeed. No matter how much power of mind you put to it, you cannot stop *being aware*.

Why? The reason is very simple.

All the power of God's Mind, which your mind shares, doesn't have the power to stop it's own awareness. *Because God cannot deny Itself*.

Awareness Is.

You have returned to a point in mind where you touch the eternal. Yes, this has merely been a guided meditation. A guided inquiry into levels of apparent reality. But, neverthe-less, it *is* part of your mind's experience. Your consciousness traveled this imaginary journey.

[—pause—]

Gently. Gently bring your awareness back into this room. Back into your human body sitting here, listening to these words. *Notice*, again, that you have been doing a meditation.

Bring your awareness to your body as you sit, right now. Just as we did at the beginning of this meditation. Notice your body sitting.

I love you. I am within you, even now. Can you tell? Where do you think this voice is coming from?

Do you really think "I-am" out here in another body? (Or, "I-am" in the words of a book?) You *know* better. My body can be laid down as easily as yours. And I will watch with you, as it is. So, my friend and fellow traveler, who am I? Who is this voice that shares this meditation with you?

"I-am" with you. Within your true self. True awareness. We are the One Child, the holy Self, together.

This true self-awareness is here, now. AMEN.

[End of Guided Meditation]

If possible, take some time to be still after completing this meditation. Open yourself to feel what it stirs up inside of you. As with the earlier practices, feel free to make this meditation your own. If the language and phrasing as offered doesn't resonate within you, please find your own. Trust your own inner knowing and imagination.

This is a healing process and, like all processes, it takes time.

Singing,

> *Amazing Grace, how sweet the sound*
> *That saved a soul like me.*
> *I once was lost, but now am found*
> *Was blind, but now I see.*

How can we come to sing this? To sing it so deeply, so intimately and personally that its truth resonates from our innermost beings? How? This is the song the Buddha sang, that Moses, Krishna, and Mohammed sang. Did you think it was only Christian? Well, my friend, it isn't. This song can't be held or designated by any way or path. It is the universal song of awakening.

We will each sing it one day. Everyone, no matter what outward form our faith. Singing,

> *Was bound, but now I'm free.*

part III

GOING DEEPER

What is to give light must endure burning.

—Viktor Frankl

Introduction

Yesterday, a friend of mine who is terminally diagnosed said, "Knowing that my life is going to end often makes me remember how precious this all is. But sometimes knowing this is so painful that I have a hard time being present and I just want to run away from it all—my death, my life, all of it."

This is the dilemma, the basic question uncovered. Is living our dying possible? Or is it too much to ask?

Sometimes it is too much to ask. Don't be ashamed. We've already mentioned the value of defense mechanisms—how they can serve us in critical situations. The journey's path is unique for each of us. And, ultimately, we learn to go deeper. This is often painful and frightening. It's as if we are literally being asked to lay down our sense of self boundary and identity.

Part of the yoke we bear in awakening to life's sacredness is a constant self-testing of our own comfort and defense boundaries. Each of the practices espoused in this book is an example of pushing up against these boundaries. We push in order to go deeper into ourselves, into our falsehoods and truths. Yes, at times we feel like we can't take another day of digging. Our morning prayer might as well be, "Please God, don't let this be another one of those learning days." This is okay, this too is part of the process.

When we can, we go deeper. Imagine life as a vast ocean. Sometimes the waves are high and rough; other times, smooth and calm. Sometimes we feel ourselves definitely swimming forward; other times we are tossed around, dunked and bobbed. This ocean-life is viewed by most of our fellow swimmers as a two-dimensional horizontal plane. Not very often do we hear stories told about the great depth of life that exists below us, deep into the ocean itself. We are taught to remain upon the water's surface. To go deep is to drown, to lose yourself. Yet in the center of our being, there is a faint voice whispering, "Go deeper, go deeper." Coming to value and honor that voice is coming to embrace the spiritual nature of life's journey. It's no accident that millions of people are now starting to hear that whisper more distinctly.

In times when I feel myself being tossed about, swept away within the ocean's current, it helps me to think of this analogy. It helps me to remember that I can go deeper than I'm currently swimming. And in the quiet deeper waters of myself, I can hear that other "voice" more clearly. Learn to go deep. Use the practices in this book and any others you can find. Seek counsel from teachers, therapists, the dying, the voice within your own heart. Swim around as deeply as you can.

And when you just can't stay so deep, that's fine

too. Float on the life preserver of denial for a while. If you are at all like me, the deeper you go, the more you'll find yourself suddenly floating in new pockets of denial. It will be surprising at first. Try not to become discouraged.

Living our dying is part of the way to the sacred. That way is cyclical. There are ups and downs, ins and outs. Going deeper, floating. Try to develop some understanding and compassion for yourself as you travel along this journey. Besides, who said that you can't do some very deep work while floating? Often we learn our biggest lessons through contrast. Times of floating can also be times of great illumination. How else could we know the depths without the surface to provide contrast? No part or experience of the journey is separate from the whole.

To go deeper is sometimes to have a hard and painful time being present. To go deeper is sometimes to want to run away from it all and float mindlessly. These are all normal, natural places to visit along the journey. I've never known anyone who's seriously embraced living our dying and not been overwhelmed at least part of the time.

I honor us and our going deeper. I honor us and our floating too. Living our dying is about coming to honor the whole journey.

More Stories, Reflections, and Practices

Dear Ron and Michael,

"I'm sorry" isn't enough, is it? I've wondered how I could feel your forgiveness for real—not in some predetermined guided visualization designed to make me feel all gushy and lovely inside, but for real. I've wondered if you have forgiven me. Maybe you can't. Maybe I can't. But where you are—heaven!, another incarnation, out there, in here, wherever that is—we're told that now, wherever you are after you've left this bodily life, is supposed to be a place of such spaciousness that forgiveness is instinctual, natural. Automatic. But I wonder . . .

In this earthly life nothing is automatic. So why am I to believe it will be any different in the next life? I hope it is. Or, rather, I hope you've both forgiven me.

I ran from your dying because I was scared of my own. I didn't know that then. Then, I thought you two were the ones who were scared. You were too fearful to embrace the spiritual truth of your all-encompassing God self. You were too afraid to leap over the edge and claim your part in God's life. I said I didn't blame you. But I did. I was like the fake Buddhist who claims to have compassion for his brother's suffering, but really feels pity. I wanted you to run away with me—off to the commune, to the spiritual community. Away from the world and into God's service. But you didn't.

You stayed behind and sometimes thought I was crazy, and other times thought you weren't good enough to "leap" like me. Well, you were farther along with AIDS, closer to your physical death than I. I see now, as my own disease progresses, that your ill bodies helped bring you back to some grounding. You couldn't wholeheartedly fool yourself like I did. Death was too close.

I'm sorry I abandoned you. I abandoned my promise that we would be together through your dying processes.

The "near-death experience" survivors say that, when we die, we go through a tunnel or some sort of metaphor of transition (it is culturally determined). Then on the other side of the passage, we meet up with all our loved ones who've died before us. They've gathered to help us continue our journey further. What I really want to say is that, when I die and travel through the tunnel, I hope you are there for me, Ron and Michael. I've thought again and again of who might be waiting for me. And I want you to know that I need you both to be waiting there, opening your hearts and arms to me.

I try to feel that opening now. Sometimes I think I do. But is it just wishful thinking? Michael laughing, tossing his head back. Or eyes wide as quarters, like that time you opened an envelope to see that Monty had given the Center a check for a thousand dollars. Or Ron announcing proudly to the group that finally, after stopping AZT, his sex drive had returned. And

Ron looking up at me with tears in his eyes as I said I'd go to the hospital with him and be there when he dies.

But I didn't go that far. I was with neither of you at your moment of death. I'd already left, a thousand miles away in a religious cult, busy finding God and eternal life, while you "nonseekers" died.

Well, I'm back now. I'm sorry. And I need your help.

Love,

Joseph

I wrote this letter at a weekly writing group I attend for people who are affected by AIDS (not just those who are HIV positive, but friends, family, healthcare workers, anyone associated or affected in any way). The exercise was to "Write a letter to someone." Even though that "someone" was not specified to be someone who was dead, most of the group that day wrote to a person who had died. It's an important practice.

The way our writing group functions is that, after the allotted writing time is up, everyone takes a turn reading aloud what they just wrote. (You can "pass" and not read aloud, of course.) When I read the above letter to the group I gained some clarity. I discovered my still unaddressed guilty feelings about a time of my life that involved my running away to a secluded spiritual community in Wisconsin. Ron and Michael were my best friends in Dallas and both were board members of a non-profit organization I'd founded. I loved them deeply and left just as they were beginning to become seriously ill. This running-away pattern was not new for me. As I read the letter aloud to the group I realized how, though I've worked a lot on forgiving the specificity of having run away from Ron and Michael then, I'm coming up against some new walls on forgiving myself for the daily running away I still sometimes do—the pattern continued in my present life. It's deep, subtle work, cutting close to the bone of growth for me. This exercise served as a trigger, inspiring me to swim into some even deeper waters than I had consciously known about.

Here are some specific practices to try in letter writing:

- Write a letter to someone you know who is dead. Be specific. If you need forgiveness from them, ask for it and remind them of why. If you need to forgive them, do the same. Come as clean as you can. Then read the letter aloud to someone if possible. If you can't, that's okay. Don't let your fear of having to read the letter aloud keep you from writing it in the first place. You can always destroy the letter without anyone else seeing it. I would suggest, however, if you aren't going to read it aloud to someone else, let it sit for a day or two and then read it aloud to yourself. Reading aloud is important. It puts some extra life-force behind your letter's intention and often reveals hidden triggers into deeper issues.

- Have someone else read aloud the letter you wrote in the practice above. Listen to it as though you were the deceased person to whom it was addressed. Hear it as that person might, with an open heart. Then write a response letter back to yourself. Try to write as the person who has died. Make it a specific response to your first letter. Let your imagination take over. When you have finished, read the letter aloud to the person who is helping you do this practice.

- Write a letter to someone who is still alive and in the process of dying. State what scares you about his or her dying and about your own. Be honest. Be specific. Ask or offer forgiveness if you need to. Don't be afraid to be emotional. Use the "d" words. In direct words, *acknowledge the fact* that you know he or she is dying. Don't skirt your fears. And, of course, if you can, send the letter. And, even better, go to the person and read it aloud if you can. As always, if you can't share the letter, this is fine too. It is quite powerful to read the letter aloud to yourself, while pretending the person to whom it's addressed is in the room hearing it with you.

- Write a letter to your friends and family from your imagined deathbed—an "as I lay dying" letter. (I did this again just last week. It's a revealing practice.) Say what you need to say. See what comes up. Do whatever you want to do with the insights that come from this practice.

Also, feel free to create your own specifics in letter-writing practice. Experiment. You can use the general principle of letter writing in any way that serves your own self-discovery.

What's Dying?

This chapter offers additional practices that can further openings into the greater journey of living our dying. Throughout this work, you may begin to notice that practices that once seemed exclusive to conscious dying are, now, equally relevant to conscious living. The definitions we once maintained between living and dying are becoming increasingly blurred. In this instance, the blurring of boundaries is progress. We are coming to an experiential realization that living and dying are indeed inseparable.

In Chapter 2, the basic practice of "seeing change, seeing dying" was introduced. This practice asks that we begin training the mind to equate *change* and *dying* as the same process. It is a form of labeling our perceptions. As we practice, our capacity for embracing the dying nature of all things grows. Simultaneously with our growing inclusion of dying into the most ordinary of life's experiences, we begin to recognize that we've been maintaining a greater illusion about life. That newly discovered greater illusion is an erroneous belief in permanence. Living our dying invites us to recognize the "illusion of permanence" in all aspects of life: our careers, relationships, belief systems, emotional states, finances, health, intellect, confidence—the list is endless. Nothing in our life is truly permanent; everything changes. When we ask, "What's dying?," the response becomes, "Everything."

Cultivating a New Way of Speaking and Listening
When I first became a chaplain the problem of how to introduce honesty into a conversation arose. At our hospital none of the chaplains wore "clergy" uniforms of any kind. We didn't wear white medical coats either. Except for our staff identification badges, we looked decidedly unlike hospital employees. The reason was simple. We didn't want to overtly introduce any "authority" issues, either medical or spiritual, into our dialogues with patients. Easing away

from the uniform that says "I'm an authority," we hoped to create a better environment for an honest sharing of the patient's feelings and concerns.

So I would enter the hospital room and introduce myself. "Hello, my name is Joseph. I'm the chaplain on this floor and I thought I'd stop by and meet you." Still pretty innocuous. I didn't look that imposing, not toting a hospital chart nor a Bible. But where does one proceed from there? It was a problem I had to consciously address.

In daily life we greet people every day. "Hello." We usually fill our greetings with what rhetoricians call "phatic" conversation. Phatic conversation is that which is merely polite. It conveys no true content and expects no real answer. "Hello, good to see you." And we never break our stride as we keep walking. This may be the rule for casual worldly contact, but it doesn't serve us when trying to be truly present and alive with someone.

I wanted to be real with the people I encountered lying in those hospital beds. I wanted to provide them with the opportunity to share their feelings about what was happening in their experience, to empower them by listening to that sharing, and to honor their process. I wanted to actually learn something about them, about life and myself. So, naturally, I thought the best way to proceed was to be direct.

"How are you feeling?" I would ask.

This was usually a mistake. It's such a trite, commonplace question. And since most of the time someone who asks this doesn't want to hear any answer but, "Fine, I'm feeling fine," that's all I would usually get in response. "Oh, I'm fine. Everything's fine." Or, if the patient were honest, she might answer, "Well, my stomach hurts due to the medication; and this tube in my arm hurts even more." Often I would be given a litany of medical problems and physical-pain sensations. When asked "How are you feeling?" most of us don't think to apply the question to our emotional lives, especially in a hospital. We answer with a list of our physical symptoms.

I spoke of this problem with my fellow chaplains. Everyone understood. It was then I was introduced to what I came to call "the Chaplain's Number One Question." Instead of asking "How do you feel?", this pastoral-care model asks: "What's this like for you?"

And a new world opened up for me. Think about it. When was the last time anyone looked you in the eyes and sincerely asked, "What's this situation you're in now really like for you? I'd like to hear about it." And then listened to what you had to say? Usually, most people we meet are busy trying to tell us what our experience is supposed to be like. This is no different in hospitals, especially with all the extra baggage of fear that accompanies death.

Truthfully asking, "What is this like for you?" is a big step toward cultivating a sincere practice of speaking and listening. As with our euphemisms for the "d" words, it is important to notice our ways of conversing. Pay attention. Begin noticing phatic statements (like "How are you doing?") that introduce closure ("Oh, I'm fine") into a conversation. Instead, try to find ways of introducing inclusiveness and openness.

As we go deeper into the inner and outer work of living our dying, language becomes increasingly important. It directly reflects our intentions toward the world around us. One way we learn to develop this more inclusive language is by noticing the words and phrases others use—particularly those of teachers, friends, and acquaintances who make us, as listeners, feel safely included and listened to. When you experience contact with such a presence, listen carefully to how he or she speaks, the inclusive nature of the words they choose. *Of course, an inner intention of inclusiveness is a prerequisite.* Just mimicking the outer form will not work. But so often our sincere intentions are masked by our functional inability to communicate those intentions effectively.

Begin to ask, "How does this make you feel?" within yourself too. *What's this like for me, now?* And take the time and compassion to listen to your own inner response. You are literally learning a new way to speak and think and relate. Be gentle; healing processes take time.

Another aspect of my own speaking that I discovered while doing this work was the subconscious desire to fix or cure everyone. At first, when someone presented me with an emotional problem, I'd respond with various solutions or suggestions designed to cheer them up, and have them look on the positive side. I was operating in the old cure-centered model. Whereas later on, in pastoral care, I was made to realize that often there is little we can do to alleviate another's emotional suffering, other than to sincerely listen. Usually, the speaker does not really want my solution, she wants someone simply to hear her out. It's an important lesson.

As we come to understand this lesson, we can begin a practice of conscious listening. In conscious listening we are "conscious" of our own inner response to what someone else is telling us. We become conscious of our desire to fit the speaker's story with a newly scripted ending of our own (usually a script that doesn't mirror to us something unpleasant like pain, death and dying). From this type of listening we listen not only to what someone else says to us, but to what our own egos are saying in reply. This is truly honoring the other person's individual process. In conscious listening there is often nothing more to reply than, "I hear you." No trying to fix, no miracle solutions, just a simple, direct, "I hear what you're saying." When we connect on this level, what more is needed?

Another trap we innocently fall into is the "I'm listening without judgment" illusion. At workshops or group meetings we often hear statements like: "During sharing, listen to what another person says without judgment." Though the intention may be sincere—to facilitate a sense of spaciousness and safety—in practical real-life application, listening without judgment is impossible to do, and it is not *conscious* listening. To begin with, we may feel nonjudgmental about what we're hearing for a time (which most likely means we're judging it as "nonthreatening"), but sooner or later we'll hear something that triggers a response in us. As human beings we naturally judge whatever our senses process into our minds. When we are instructed, "Don't judge," functionally we're being asked to ignore, repress, or deny our natural thought processes. Therefore, usually in trying to obey the teacher's instructions of nonjudgment, we add another wall between ourselves and others. A more conscious approach to listening would be the advice: "When listening to someone, notice your own judgments as they arise. Notice your feelings about what the other person is saying. Don't try to deny your rising thoughts and judgments, but don't believe them either. Just notice what your ego-mind is saying, notice the same old scripts and patterns the ego tries to get you to obey." As pointed out earlier, conscious listening means we are "conscious" of our own inner responses as well as of outer stimuli. We note what's happening to ourselves within, cultivating awareness of the *inner response*, without spinning off into an *egoic reaction*. It's just more grist for the mill of personal awakening. Here we approach what might be called "conscious thinking."

These are only a few general examples of how we must begin to rethink the ways in which we speak and listen to one another. And they are not formulas. We can say "I hear you" or "What's this like for you?" all day long, but if we don't truly mean it, we are not honestly practicing. Ultimately we return to our intention and willingness to open, change, and grow—which is also willingness to be confronted by our own ego games and attachments. This is the work we must do.

Seeking Comfort

I spent the majority of my life thinking that my real purpose as a human being was to avoid pain as much as possible, and to just try to get comfortable. I don't think there's ever been a person born who didn't see life in that way, at least for a time. Comfort is a definite goal in most of our lives.

As I studied and immersed myself in various spiritual traditions, I began to see the misunderstanding of "seeking comfort." If I sought comfort first and foremost, I could indeed avoid pain a good deal of the time. I could protect myself from suffering and life's unpleasantness as much as possible. Again, many people would ask, "What's wrong with trying to avoid pain in your life? Are you crazy or something?" But let's remember that the world of the seeker often seems crazy or inverted to the nonseeker.

The problem with seeking comfort is, by doing so, we cannot look upon the here and now with openness. Rather, we look upon the here and now through controlling eyes. "How can I avoid *this* and get to something more comfortable." And if we are dedicated to comfort no matter what, when we come up against pain of any kind, we are going to turn the other way. Part of taking another look is coming to see pain differently. Pain is not something bad or negative, to be avoided at all costs. Pain is another tool, another route by which we travel in this journey.

For the Christian apologist C. S. Lewis, pain was God's chisel. In Lewis' analogy, the human condition is a block of uncut stone and God, the Master Sculptor, chisels away with pain at our ego-stone in order to perfect us. Thus our suffering becomes virtuous, a movement toward holiness. An action of perfection. This view is helpful to me, but I personally can't accept the idea that God is "responsible" for my life's pain (even if it is for my own good). I've resolved my doubts by taking Lewis' premise and joining it with a more Buddhist notion: life is painful and we suffer not by divine plan, but because pain is simply part of life's curriculum while here in body. For me this view retains the understanding that life's pain serves an invaluable function by chipping away at our unfinished rock, at our ego eggshell, while removing God as the personal Dispenser of Pain. In this understanding, pain is not "given" by God but is instead a part of human growth that's as natural as aging, for example. (Also, the imagery of a hard stone being worn smooth by a river's constant flow is more to my liking than that of a sculptor chipping away, because there's no "God" doing painful things to us, only the life-river's natural flow and movement.) In either metaphor, however, bit by bit we are worn away to a newborn self beneath. In our taking another look at pain—which includes injustice, hate, fear, all the mental and emotional pain of life as well as the physical—we can begin to see a context for pain being something to embrace, instead of something to escape.

We learn so much through our suffering. Yes, it's painful. Yes, we want it to be over. But it is *here*, regardless. It is part of our life. We feel it. And the amazing thing that every expert who works with pain tells us is that, once we stop trying to resist our pain, it literally changes texture. Often the pain seems to lessen in intensity. Yet even if it doesn't lessen, the pain nevertheless transforms into something other than "useless, meaningless" suffering. From here, we can begin to understand pain's larger role in our spiritual development.

More clearly than anything else I know, pain teaches us about *attachment*. The Indian saint Ramana Maharshi spent the final months of his life in great pain. He had terminal cancer and his pain was so intense that it would often cause him to scream out at night, disturbing the entire community. Many of his students were unsure of what to make of this. Certainly, they thought, such an enlightened master wouldn't feel pain and die from such a common disease as cancer. Trying to form a rationale, one of his students said to him, "Perhaps you don't feel the pain?" Ramana's reply was instructive, "There is pain, but there is no suffering." Of course Ramana still felt the pain, so much so it made him scream and wince in agony. Yet he claimed, "There is no suffering." From our Western-minded perspective we might ask, "What could he mean by that? What's the difference between suffering and pain?"

To go deeper into this question we need to begin by acknowledging that everyone, the enlightened being and the nonenlightened alike, feels pain. Pain is a normal physical or emotional occurrence. We feel physical pain when we cut our finger and we feel emotional pain when a friend is angry at us. It is a mistake to think that the aim of spirituality is to eradicate pain. In the Christian tradition we need look no further than Jesus; his life was filled with pain, as were the lives of many of Christianity's greatest saints. But unlike pain, suffering (in the sense that Ramana Maharshi was referring to it) is neither physical nor emotional. In Ramana's way of looking at the world, the root of suffering is *mental*. We suffer because, in our minds, we are *attached* to certain ideas of *how life ought to be*. We want things a certain way—"my way." And when we don't get things the way we want them in life, we feel the separation between "what really is" and "what we would rather it be." This attachment to how life *should* be is originally mental. From the mind it extends to affect all aspects of our experience. We emotionally feel pain because we're not happy with life as it is. We can also physically internalize or somatize this pain so that we feel it in our bodies: stress, ulcers, some heart conditions, to name a few. Yet still, the root cause of this type of suffering is within our own minds, our own mental attachment to things *being other* than they are.

In Ramana Maharshi's example, he was feeling the immense physical pain that often accompanies cancer. Yet he was able to say truthfully that "I am not suffering" because he wasn't attached to his life being other than for what it was. He wasn't clinging to comfort. Of course, he didn't enjoy the pain and would have been relieved to see it go. *But he didn't mentally run away from the "what is" of his life—the pain of dying from cancer.* He lived his pain and dying, using the moments of his life as a vehicle for his continued awakening. Ramana was Hindu. Yet this idea that "attachment brings about suffering" is hardly exclusive to Hinduism. In the Second Noble Truth, Buddha taught that the cause of suffering is our mental attachment. We cling to this or that idea about how our life should be. In doing this, we miss the very "what is" before us. To end this suffering, Buddha taught, we need only to stop clinging to our attachments. (Of course this is easier said than done, but nevertheless it is the way beyond suffering.) And this instruction is hardly exclusive to Eastern spirituality. In the Judeo-Christian tradition, letting go of attachment is called "surrendering to God's will."

Physical and emotional pain teaches us intimately about the difficulty in truly surrendering. When we feel pain, we want it to go away. In this culture particularly, we've become very attached to life being without pain. But what if we take another look at pain and begin to see it as a natural process of life? What if we begin to see our physical and emotional pain as life's teaching tools, as fingers pointing toward our attachments and nonsurrendered desires and ideas? From this new perspective, the question of "Do I deserve this pain?" cannot arise. Pain is not a matter of "deserving it." Pain simply is part of life's expression and ongoing process—part of our learning situation. The question then becomes, "Can I live my life fully while experiencing this pain? Can I let go of my attachment to a 'comfortable' life, and to the ideal I have in my mind about just what that life should look like? Can I, instead, snuggle into my life experience as it actually is right here and now?"

But why? Why do this? Why not just seek comfort and avoid pain *while also* trying to cultivate the sacred?

The answer we never really want to hear is: it is impossible to seek *both* comfort and the sacred whole of life's experience. Seeking comfort is a matter of control and manipulation—of "I know what I want." Seeking the sacred life is a matter of letting go and surrender—of "Not my will but Thine be done." One is a matter of holding on and aligning with our egoic wants and desires; the other is surrender, opening, and letting go. It is impossible to simultaneously cling and let go. As the fourteenth-century Christian mystic Meister Eckhart wrote, "Some people want to recognize God only in some pleasant enlightenment—and then they get pleasure and enlightenment but not God." For most of us, this is a radically different way of looking at pain's role in life. It is also a radically new look at what it means to "live the good life."

How simple it would be to make pain versus suffering into a spiritually correct formula. A man dying of cancer explained plainly that "I'm not going to suffer." After unsuccessful attempts to control his cancer, his doctors gave up, giving him a prognosis of two months or less to live. He was not the least bit fearful, he said. Though he hadn't yet experienced great physical pain in his process, he knew that when he did, when the final stages of his cancer began in earnest, he would clearly recognize the difference between pain and suffering. Since he was Buddhist, he said, he knew the difference. The more he talked and the more he asserted (almost evangelically) that "I am not going to suffer," the more obvious his fear became. He was too sure of himself. There was no humility, no room for honesty. For him, the opposition of suffering versus pain had become the Answer to which he clung. His understanding was intellectual, not experiential. He'd embraced a formula he thought would protect him from suffering.

Though we may be able to bypass or deny life's pain and suffering for a time, eventually, every formula will fail to work. Living our dying is not about finding the right formula. It would be more accurate to say that living our dying is about finding that the *only* formula is the Formula of Being Authentically Who You Are at the Moment. But this is no formula. You get nothing from it other than being who you are. Nothing changes outside of you. You simply become more aware.

This formula of being authentically who you are is the spirit in which I encourage you to do the practices outlined in this book. Remember, none of the living-our-dying practices are formulas; they are only tools. On one hand, authenticity of *being* is all-important; but on the other, *doing* is essential as well. Being and doing need not be opposites. Do the practices. But keep an awareness of yourself as you do them.

And one more note: I am not saying that the spiritually correct position is to avoid the temporary comfort of pain medication. Certain spiritual traditions, particularly some schools of Buddhism, are quite strict with this. They teach that any drug-induced alteration of consciousness (including the lessening of pain) fogs the person's ability to rest in "clear mind"—which, in some traditions, is particularly important as one nears the moment of death. My personal opinion is that a great distance exists between "seeking comfort as a life goal" and taking pain medication to improve the quality, even awareness, of life along the journey. When asked about the theological problem of pain medication, a Buddhist priest dying of AIDS put it this way: "I don't want to hear about all that 'clear-mind-no-drugs' talk. I don't even want to hear it. That's not the mind we're talking about. The mind we're talking about when we say 'clear mind' isn't affected by a little morphine."

Letting Be, First

Often I hear someone who's referring to a problem say, "I just let go of it." But usually what is meant by this is, "I just closed my mind to this problem so it will hopefully go away." My experience is that before we can "let go," we've got to be able to just "let be." If we are not content first to just let things be, we are usually still attached to the problem working out one way or the other. And attachment is *not* the essence of letting go. If we let be—just be here, right now—we'll find out if we have any secret grasping attachments. In this way we can come to see the root cause of our suffering in the situation. After we've "let be" for a while, then we naturally come to letting go. This authentic letting go happens without our *doing* it.

When we say "let go," what are we really saying? Let go of what? In one way of looking at it, we are letting go of the lie. It is the lie that says, if we "hold on," life can be controlled. It is the lie that says that we can prevent change (which is often painful) from happening in our lives. We can hold, fixate, even stop life's flow. We can defend ourselves against the changing, decaying, growing, birthing, dying process of life. This is the lie we each tell ourselves until we learn otherwise. Holding on is a temporary illusion. It doesn't work in the long run. In our hearts, each of us knows this. All of the spiritual traditions that I'm aware of say the same thing: the Way is to let go, to surrender. Try *letting be* first and see what happens.

The Joining of Intentions

A conscious joining of intentions on the "fellow soul-traveler" plane is important for those of us who are endeavoring to live our dying. (We spoke of this plane of consciousness as the first of the "higher channels" in Chapter 4, "The Self That Doesn't Die.") And this joining is likewise important for us on levels of reality higher than the soul-traveler plane, as well. This process might be thought of as a joining of intentions with the "will of God" or with the "universal unfolding."

In some traditions, we are talking about nothing more than conscious and sincere prayer. Though I pray daily, often hourly or more, for our purposes here I prefer to speak of prayer in other terms, because many people have a lot of connotative baggage that accompanies "prayer" and "praying." To avoid this baggage for now, I suggest we consider a more accurate and less charged word: "alignment." In the process of alignment we ask that our own individual intentions be aligned with (1) our souls' highest good and (2) the universal unfolding of all life or God's will.

This type of spiritual work needs to be done consciously and conscientiously. Often I ask people if they've prayed and the response is something like, "Sure, I always want this to be for the highest good of everyone involved." But that was not the question. Knowing a spiritual principle of "highest good" is not the same thing as actually stopping for a moment, and taking the time and effort to actively surrender our egoic will to a higher soul-centered will. For any spiritual practice to work, we've got to actually *practice* the practices, not just know about them intellectually. C. S. Lewis once said that "to offer the world instruction on prayer would be impudence." He believed that our relationship with the divine is too highly individualistic and personal for the generalizations necessary in a "how to" instruction. This resonates as good advice to me and so I'm not going to try to tell you exactly "how to" align. I am, however, going to share some important pointers that I've discovered for myself as I've endeavored to more fully live my own dying. Perhaps these pointers will resonate for you. I know they help me. What follows is what might be called my primary alignment or prayer—the one I find myself saying most often in my life today. It's a little different every time I say it. At this moment, it is:

Dear God,
I do not ask for any change in the outer circumstances or in "what is." I'm asking only that, *through these circumstances*, I will come to love my brothers and sisters even more. So I can come to know them as You do, God.
Help me see this through Your Eyes.
Help me join on a soul-level with all I meet.
Help me have courage, softness, and vulnerability.
For this "I thirst" and for nothing more.
May Your will be done on earth, as It is in heaven.
Amen.

Occasionally I like to add "I thirst" at the closing of the prayer since, according to the Gospels, these were the last words Jesus Christ spoke upon the cross. It resonates within me. Also adding the line from the traditional Lord's Prayer connects me to my childhood spiritual roots and sense of depth within myself, as well as to the greater tradition of Christianity throughout the ages. Feel free to use these lines in your moments of prayer and alignment, but also feel free to find your own special phrases that likewise resonate powerfully for you. Here's another possibility, something like:

Dear God,
I'm asking only to recognize Your grace and perfec-

tion in this situation. And if I can't, help me to be open
to accepting the mystery before my eyes.

Amen.

Remember that aligning our intentions upon a soul-centered level is an ongoing act throughout the day. As Marianne Williamson writes in *Illuminata*, "Each morning, or
any time you are about to go anywhere or do anything, go
over the scenario in your mind. Pray, consciously, that the
circumstance in question be used for the purposes of love,
that God's rays of light might shine upon it."

Again, one of the reasons I use the word "alignment" is to avoid the supplicating aspect sometimes associated with prayer. Notice my sample alignments do not ask
for anything to be "handled" or "changed" outwardly by
God. At this depth of prayer, I feel that it is a misunderstanding for me to tell God what is best for my awakening.
Besides, I'm usually asking for what my ego desires for its own
self-maintenance. This is what Oscar Wilde was hinting at
when he quipped, "When the gods want to punish us,
they answer our prayers." In these alignments, I think it is
important to undo our egoic wishes for control that have
for so long dominated much of our prayer life. This is why
I suggest beginning by emphasizing something akin to "I
do not ask for a change in the outer circumstances."

Here I would like to reiterate the reason I think of
this higher joining of intention as "alignment," instead
of prayer. Many of us have profoundly intimate ways of
connecting with God that definitely involve supplicating
prayer (Mother Teresa comes immediately to mind). It
would be impudence for me to advise you to stop or change

your practice in regard to prayer. Rather, consider this an introduction to an *additional* practice of alignment with holy intentions.

Undoing Specialness

We human beings spend a great deal of time and effort trying to set ourselves off as special from one another. Nevertheless, in God's eyes and in the awakened perception of sacred self, no one of us is more special than another. We are all God's beloved children. Sometimes as I write or speak to groups, I can feel myself edging toward specialness. "Ours is a special disease. My suffering is greater!" It took me years to realize how being special is a trap.

At first I thought my having been diagnosed with a terminal disease obviously made me special. After all, wasn't I more interested in addressing the bigger questions of life because of my special terminal status? I was different, I thought. I really knew what it was like to live upon life's edge. Since, I've come to see how this reasoning was a fiction I told myself. It served me well, because I didn't want to embrace my dying seriously yet. The specialness I coveted for my diagnosis served as a powerful way to keep my dying at arm's length. I didn't have to *live* my dying when I could milk it for its dramatics, for its special star quality (and, remember, the show's star never dies). Being special for being a "long-term survivor," for being a writer, a spokesperson for spiritual awakening through illness—all these things were my little perks of specialness I thought I deserved. As I've become more intimate with myself, I'm watching my desire to be someone special resurface again and again. It's part of the work in living our dying. We begin to cultivate our ordinariness, our basic sense that we are not different nor special from others.

In Zen this concept of ordinariness is called "nothing special." In Christianity we find it exemplified by the spiritual practice of humility—not a false humility, but a deep humbling before God, life's unfolding, and life's perfection. From the higher channels of perception, we can see life's process and pain in just this way. We see souls on a greater learning adventure that extends far before and after the body's birth and death. To glimpse into this reveals the absurdity of maintaining specialness for ourselves, our chosen few friends, and family.

I'm mentioning this now because specialness is one of the most delicious traps of conscious-dying work: we feel ourselves special, almost noble, because we're willing to confront the bigger questions and fears in life. But it is a trap, nonetheless. Ultimately specialness separates us from others, which is not the essence of living our dying, or opening our heart.

The Underlying Practice

Perhaps the underlying practice is simply openness. Openness to your own feelings, emotions, and thoughts. Openness to the feelings of others, to situations, to the "what is" you find before you in today's life-classroom. It is also the underlying preparation for being alive with yourself as you die. American Buddhist nun Pema Chödrön writes,

> If your everyday practice is to open to all your emotions, to all the people you meet, to all the situations you encounter, without closing down, trusting that you can

do that—then that will take you as far as you can go. And then you'll understand all the teachings that anyone has ever taught.

Enough said. Openness is a feeling—an experience—not a concept or theory. There is nothing new to write or say "about" opening. Opening is something we each must *do* for ourselves. Enough said. Time to practice. Enough said.

To begin depriving death of its greatest advantage over us, . . . let us deprive death of its strangeness, let us frequent it, let us get used to it; let us have nothing more often in mind than death. . . . We do not know where death awaits us: so let us wait for it everywhere. To practice death is to practice freedom.

—MICHEL DE MONTAIGNE

chapter 6

The Mirror: Being Alive with Someone As They Die

Today, for the first time in over four years, I spoke with an old friend of mine. Through the grapevine I'd heard he was sick, had lost a lot of weight, and looked as if he were dying. So I took a chance that the phone number I had was still good and called. Craig answered.

We spoke for maybe a quarter of an hour. Craig was still much the same person I remembered. He hadn't embarked on any conscious spiritual quest, and I didn't tell him about mine. I listened a lot. Asked questions about old friends we'd both known. We talked about symptoms and disability. Both of the Chinese pugs were fine, still fat as ever. And I told him I've always loved him and I'm thinking of him a lot lately. Next month, I'm passing through Dallas on my way to visit my parents and I'm going to stop by Craig's apartment, see him, really look at him, and take him in as deeply as I can. This scares me. On the phone, just hearing his voice, I could pretend somewhat (but not too much, his voice did sound frail and weak). In person, I'll have to be there with him for real, see his dying body for real. This scares me. The only walls separating us will be of our own making.

So I'm going to be watching my wall building. I'm going to try to be aware and careful and soft and gentle with myself and Craig. Of course, I have to let him have his walls if he wants. But I really need to let mine down now. It's time. This is my prayer for today.

After I hung up the phone, I cried for twenty minutes. Now, I wonder if I will have the courage to cry with Craig face to face? Will I let down that wall? Will he? I don't know. If I can't cry, or it isn't appropriate, that's okay. No predetermined scripts here. Just acceptance. How can I accept Craig's dying, if I can't accept my own process, walls and all? But I do want so much more. I can no longer fake it and say that I don't care about going beyond those walls.

Death comes with a lot of extra baggage in our culture, dark images and symbols that energize our deepest fears. Sometimes that baggage can be so overwhelming that we actually miss being alive with the person who is dying. We can become so swept away by our fears that we're not present at all. Instead, we are elsewhere in our mind, reacting and relating from a place behind impenetrable walls, a place of seeming safety and protection from death's dark power.

These walls appear in many different forms. One of the most common disguises itself as "spirituality." Resting in our spiritual certainty, we may feel protected from the almost unbearable pain of watching someone we love die. Another wall disguises itself as "being tough" or "holding it all together." Another wall is blatant denial, like "When you get out of this hospital . . ." Another calls itself "work." Of course there are all the drugs: alcohol, pot, sedatives, Prozac, television, caffeine, you name it. Usually we mix and match our walls. Have you ever gone to the hospital to see someone who might be dying and spent much of the time staring up at the television set, watching a soap opera you've never seen before, talking only during the commercial breaks about the most recent developments on CNN? Perhaps this is an extreme example, but then again . . .

In working with dying we must come to recognize our walls for what they are, and not dismiss them as mere moments of awkwardness or discomfort. We must be willing to courageously push through. Recognizing our walls for what they are is the first, necessary step toward being alive with someone as they are dying. And make no mistake, these are prison walls. They keep us locked within ourselves, separated from one another, our world, and God.

Nakedness

What can we really offer someone who is deep into the process of dying? What can we offer—not as healthcare workers, husbands, wives or lovers, parents or children— what can we offer as fellow beings on a journey of awakening, as fellow soul-travelers temporarily occupying these bodies while going through our own living/dying processes? What can we *do* from this larger place in our being?

After sincerely working with this question for some

time in both clinical and personal situations, the best answer I've come to is something I heard from conscious-dying advocate Ram Dass: *All I can really do is create a spacious environment within my own mind that allows someone else to die as he or she needs to die.* This is an act of consciously stepping back and listening. How else can I truly honor and learn from the person dying? When I feel myself wanting to control the process, change it, heal it or whatever, I try to become conscious of my assertions and watch my own control issues at work. The real gift I can give is to be authentically present and nonmanipulative.

This may seem confusing in light of the focus in pastoral care to "elicit the emotional process." Though I have made some very directive moves with people when working from a pastoral-care or therapeutic model, eliciting the emotional process is usually not my focus with someone who is in the last stages of the dying process. Still, there are no hard-and-fast rules. I've found if I elicit with an attitude of questioning and exploration, I am generally on safe ground. It's when I think I know just "where" the dying person needs to go next along his or her emotional and spiritual journey that I get lost in the forest of ego games.

And, of course, even the best pastoral-care model has its limitations too. Finally, we each have to go beyond our models and just sit naked with someone who is dying. If we're naked enough, the dying person's nakedness will touch ours and we'll both return to the Garden of Eden— connecting with each other in a space that's pure and open and real. Often the dying person will be in that space already, especially as he nears the moment of death. As Cicely Saunders, founder of the modern hospice movement, wrote: "The dying have shed the masks and superficialities of everyday living and they are all the more open and sensitive because of this. They see through all unreality. I remember one man saying, 'No, no reading. I only want what is in your mind and in your heart.'" It is our job to be receptive to what the dying person wants to share: his depth or his denial. I've found that by creating a spacious environment within my mind that allows another person to die as he or she needs to, I open myself for that naked contact.

This is the prime directive for death-and-dying work with another person: *I have no moral right to say how anyone should die*. If he wants to be in denial, so be it. If she wants to be angry, so be it. It is my lesson to keep my heart open and seek a higher truth within myself, but not to enforce an outward determination of what I think that truth should look like for someone else.

And, yes, strangers are easier. Of course, the more we know and love someone, the harder it is to keep this attitude of nonattachment and openness. Nevertheless, that is the lesson before us, the work we have to do. Go as far as you can and when you can't go any farther, that's okay too. You are on a journey and are learning along every step of the way.

There is another reason it is important for us to keep a spaciousness within our minds that allows another person to die as they need to die. Only in the clarity of our own nonjudgment, compassion, and nakedness can we notice the mirror the dying person holds up before us. Being with someone who is dying is like looking into a very clear and detailed mirror of our own individual process. If we have the understanding, courage, and patience with ourselves, we can see our own fears, defenses, guilt, anger, attachments, desires—all of it—surface to the foreground of this living mirror.

When I visit with someone who is dying, I try to continually check in with my own feelings and thoughts. I listen to myself. When speaking to a family member, I catch myself wanting to use euphemisms for death. I watch as my mouth sometimes utters the most amazingly inane things—as I fill up the silence in the room to avoid my own extra baggage of fear. Not too long ago, I found myself chattering with a dying man's mother, not because I was afraid of his dying, but I was afraid of *her experiencing* his dying. She wanted to bypass her own pain and I was more than willing to assist. What a mirror this was of my issues about "protecting" my own parents from the grief and pain of my dying process.

Our life experience is made of constant change. Our physical health changes. Our moods change. Our intellectual knowledge, the people whose company we keep, our desires, all change. Even our beliefs about God, death, and dying change. So far I've found only one thing that has remained throughout: the mirror before me. Yes, what the mirror reflects is changing constantly, but the mirror itself—the nature of mirrorness—is always here before me. Everywhere I turn, the mirror. I may ignore it, deny it, even curse it; but still everywhere I turn, the mirror. What a powerful realization this can be if we let it sink beneath our mental concepts and into our emotional hearts and bodies. Everywhere we turn, the mirror.

There's always more to learn. Our work with ourselves becomes subtler and subtler. Accept the gift from the person who is being a mirror for you. Only in this way can we honor the mirror for who he or she is—a part of ourselves.

Letting the Script Be

At least a dozen people were gathered. David's mother and father down from Tulsa, his sister, two nurses, and a mixture of other friends. David lay unconscious in his bed. Most of the twelve were gathered in the room around him.

David's ex-lover and best friend, Paul, had called me only an hour before. "David's about to die. You've got to come now. We're calling everybody." Since it was near five o'clock, I'd driven all the way up to suburban north Dallas via surface streets; the freeway had been out of the question. Once I arrived it did not take long to realize that the whole experience didn't really feel as if David's moment of death was at hand. How can I explain this?

Some of the usual signs of impending death were absent. No labored, rasping breaths that echo, pushing and pulling themselves throughout the house. None of his body's orifices were leaking fluids. His body seemed at peace, almost as if quietly sleeping. No shadow of pain upon his face. I looked at David, then looked at everyone else gathered in the room. They don't have a clue, I thought. It gets much worse than this. Dying from AIDS usually isn't this pretty.

The room was smothered with roses and mixed bouquets. Paul had read that it was best to try to create a sacred space in the dying room, decorating it with holy objects, candles, flowers, and incense as much as possible. At least forty candles from votive size to sticks as wide as pineapples, all lit, filled the house with varied fragrances. The air hung thick with the sweet incense and wax soot. Soft, ethereal New Age music whispered in from the living-room stereo. Everything was clearly arranged. It was time. David's supposed to die now.

I sat at the foot of the bed and tried not to judge the scene. I wanted to give David the spaciousness to die in the way he wanted. After all, this was David's house, these were his friends and family, New Age spirituality was his chosen belief system. I reminded myself that death brings out everyone's defense mechanisms so clearly. During these times we wear them as plainly as a sweater. And always there is a battle for control. The control here was in the timing. It was easy to have compassion for Paul and the parents. Of course, they wanted David's dying to be over. They wanted David to die right here in this lovely room, wanted him to die in as little pain as possible, serenely, peacefully. They didn't want to see him suffer and didn't want to feel their own pain while watching him die. Who would? So it was easy to have compassion for them. But as far as the rest of the people gathered, my patience was waning. It was obvious that the script of how David was to die had been written.

And there was a lot of jockeying for control in the room, to determine just who was to be the script's final interpreter. "What a beautiful lesson this is for Paul," a woman intoned into the room while waving an amethyst crystal over David's body like a magic wand.

"Right," I thought sarcastically, "it's all Paul's lesson. Why don't you just plaster another spiritual smile over it all and bypass your own pain some more. What about *your* lesson, Lady?" The longer I stayed, the more my compassion and tolerance seemed to be smothered by the incense and candle smoke. (What I didn't think at the time was to ask, "What about *my* lesson with this lady and all her spiritually escapist control?" This would come later.)

Several of those gathered repeatedly told David to "Go to the light; now's the time." The what-a-beautiful-lesson lady moved herself to the far corner of the room and began focusing her attention upon her crystal so "I'll be clear enough to guide David's soul on to the light." Someone announced how they'd been astrally traveling with David for the last two days and that he was extremely happy and ready to leave his body, so we needn't worry or feel sad about his dying. "Don't feel sad about this," she told us, smiling. "David told me he doesn't want that. He said, 'It's a time of great joy and celebration.'"

"He's traveling with me now," another self-proclaimed astral traveler announced. At which someone else corrected, "No, David is not completely traveling without his body, because part of his consciousness is holding on here, in his right hand." David had been a well-known visual artist, after all. These comments were followed by various people telling David he could "let go" of his right hand. The scene became more and more controlling as time passed. At one point I felt someone crouching behind me on the bed, moving or brushing at the air around my shoulders. I turned, giving this middle-aged, blonde-haired woman, wearing only white, a confused stare that said, "What are you doing?"

"I'm dusting your angel wings," she whispered.

All this continued. Everyone was busy doing their predetermined spiritual shtick and mostly ignoring David except to tell him to "go to the light." But before I left, David did awake from his unconsciousness. When his eyes opened, several people actually said, "No, David, go the other way! Toward the light! Toward the light!" Just whose pain were we avoiding?

As far as I could tell, none of us openly questioned the intention of trying to force David on along to "the other side." We did not question our own motives for this control. I soon excused myself and said good-bye to David. He was conscious and recognized who I was. That was Sunday afternoon. David didn't die until the early hours of Friday morning. The last three days of David's life the house was filled with the sound of gasping breaths and gurgling body fluids.

Our experience with David that day had many lessons. To begin with, it demonstrates how we are not in control of death's timetable no matter how hard we wish, pray, meditate, chant or scream to God that we want to be. Mostly it is a story of blinding control and the avoidance of pain masquerading as spirituality. David was a great teacher that day. What struck me most, however, was his refusal to die on cue.

Many stories seem to circulate in spiritual circles

about how the spiritually evolved die on cue. These stories are often about Hindu saints or, particularly, Tibetan lamas. The *Tibetan Book of the Dead* even goes as far as to describe how people die differently according to their degree of progress along the spiritual ladder (at the top is a sort of mystical smile, outward breath, and, with little or no pain, *presto!*, while at the unenlightened bottom is a person agonizing in pain and fear). If there is one thing that a sincere and mature spiritual seeker learns along the journey, it is to be wary of such formulas (no matter how respected the source). I know we Westerners prefer to extol the traps and prejudices in our own Judeo-Christian tradition, while turning a blind eye to the traditions of the East. But the fact is some practices, teachings, and traditions within Buddhism, Hinduism, and so forth, plainly exist to maintain the authority of the "priest class" and its organized religious hierarchy. Of course, in every tradition there are enlightened individuals who transcend the system while still teaching and working within it. It is easy to criticize Christianity for its blatant abuses of authoritarianism when it comes to the Way, but those canards and abuses are found in all traditions regardless of geographic or theological origin.

Let me return to the point at hand: dying on cue, according to a predetermined script. Sometimes this happens, but usually there is little to be learned from such a death experience. Since dying involves a great deal of teaching and learning for all involved, it's no wonder that the predetermined scripts get tossed. How are we going to really learn and grow if everything goes just the way we want it? The lesson I've experienced over and over is to let go of *my imagined script*. It is a lesson of opening to the real scene as it actually is, not what we'd rather it be. In spiritual circles so often we maintain predetermined scripts of what we're supposed to feel and how an experience is supposed to be. We substitute "spiritual correctness" for honesty of heart. But what if we kept another model of dying in mind? Remember the courageous honesty of Zen master Suzuki Roshi when he said on his deathbed, "I do not want to die." He didn't fake it, not even for spiritual appearances. Suzuki knew of a higher truth than appearances, the integrity of self-honesty toward this moment of experience.

In Suzuki's example, there is no predetermined script of "how" to die, only an injunction to try to be as honest as possible. This is not about outer appearance, but inner awareness. During his final days with cancer, he called his students together and said:

> If when I die, the moment I'm dying, if I suffer that is all right, you know; that is suffering Buddha. No confusion in it. Maybe everyone will struggle because of the physical agony or spiritual agony, too. But that is all right, that is not a problem.

It is not a problem because there is no spiritually correct script that must be followed in order to enter the kingdom of heaven. No path to follow here, just honesty. Just awareness of what is. Just self-honesty. Our greater suffering comes from not allowing the script to unfold the way it is. Nothing in Earthly life is perfect. Life just is. Our emotional health is not perfect, our physical health is not perfect, our relationships are certainly not perfect. Yet, if we insist upon masquerading perfection, we will miss being alive with our family, friends, and even our very selves, as we lie dying. Suzuki went on to tell his students, "We should be grateful to have a limited body . . . like mine, like yours. If you had a limitless life [on Earth,] it would be a real problem for you."

Care versus Cure

Living our dying also asks us to dismiss the old-fashioned notion that our goal is to "cure" ourselves. "A major difference between care and cure," writes Thomas Moore in *Care of the Soul*, "is that cure implies the end of trouble. If you are cured, you don't have to worry about whatever was bothering you any longer. But care has a sense of ongoing attention. There is no end." To release our attachment to fixing, to ending, to "getting it over and done with," is to release our grasping for control. Often, when working with someone who is in the final process of dying, we quickly embrace the cure model, which in this case would be death. As pointed out in the story of David's dying, we can fall into the trap of wanting to cure the problem of dying with a controlled, scripted death. It's no coincidence that death has been called the "ultimate cure."

A care-centered approach, on the other hand, asks us to embrace a "sense of ongoing attention" that requires no easy black-and-white formulas. No answers or solutions. It demands nakedness and a willingness to open up to life's mystery. And since the process is ongoing, ongoing even beyond the death of the person, it is necessarily self-reflective *to us* who cared for and survived the person who has died. Whereas cure is something that is done *to someone else*, care is a two-way street. As I care for you, I am cared for in return. Care is a dynamic relationship and is therefore living. Care has a life of its own, a soul that's intangible and difficult to pigeonhole. When we open ourselves to really care for another person, we initiate responsibilities, acknowledging that our time, energy, and presence are of value. Also, when we care, we open ourselves to interpersonal pain and to the loss we will undoubtedly feel when the person we care for dies. In caring, we will encounter our own feelings of pain and often helplessness; we will encounter the sacred paradox of human impermanence. It's no surprise, then, that the medically based model, which sees the world only through a body-personality plane (channels 1 and 2), has so steadfastly chosen cure over care. Cure encourages no self-reflection, only evaluation as to outward success or failure.

Most people who've spent any time in the hospital are familiar with the medical/cure model. If to "cure" is the goal, death is our enemy (until death is so inevitable and the quality of life so miserable, then paradoxically, as mentioned earlier, death becomes the new cure). In the cure approach to medicine and psychotherapy, body and personality make up the totality of being. Anything else is left to the domain of clergy or soothsayer. This was evident to me from my experiences as a hospital chaplain, where more than once the value of pastoral *care* was belittled by cure-centered practitioners. Only recently, after many hospitals have discontinued their pastoral-care programs because of budget reductions, is the value of pastoral care being seriously reconsidered. Pastoral care, which is care for the soul, doesn't fare well in a culture that values productivity measurable only in concrete numbers. Like all forms of care, pastoral care is an art.

There is also a deeper teaching that care invites us to embrace. It might be called "embracing the shadow," an often paradoxical and sacred holism we each need to cultivate. According to psychologist Thomas Moore, the care-centered approach,

> appreciates the mystery of human suffering and does not offer the illusion of a problem-free life. It sees every fall into ignorance and confusion as an opportunity to discover that the beast residing at the center of the labyrinth is also an angel. . . . The Greeks told the story of the minotaur, the bull-headed flesh-eating man who lived in the center of the labyrinth. He was a threatening beast, and yet his name was Asterion—Star. I often think of this paradox as I sit with someone with tears in her eyes, searching for some way to deal with a death, a divorce, or a depression. It is a beast, this thing that stirs in the core of her being, but it is also the star of her innermost nature. We have to care for this suffering with extreme reverence so that, in our fear and anger at the beast, we do not overlook the star.

Living our dying asks us to see both the beast and the angel, within others and ourselves. To begin this new way of seeing, we become aware of our control-based self that wants to write its own predetermined script of our experience. We learn to let the script be, reminding ourselves that a one-sided cure is not the goal. Rather, we seek mutual care.

Let's look at some of the other practices and principles that a care-centered approach to living and dying might advocate: feeling empathy; connecting beyond the costume;

accepting the paradox of pain and grace; softening; and grieving. This is not an exhaustive list (no such list exists). These
practices are, however, a good foundation from which to go
deeper. And like the other practices in this book, these too
can be misused. In working with such clear mirrors as those
who are nearing death, the fear is more clearly seen and so
more powerfully felt. As always, be gentle with yourself. There
are no answers, here. Only suggestions, possibilities.

Empathy
In the cure-centered model, it is generally considered best
to keep an emotional distance between a medical prac-
titioner and patient. But for those of us willing to live our
dying, we must dismiss such warnings from a system that,
above all else, doesn't want to look into the living mirror
before us.

When visiting someone who is deep into the dying
process, I try to open my mind and heart to touch within
myself the feelings that he or she might be feeling. Since
dying brings up our defense mechanisms, quite often the
dying person has spent little or no time with someone who
is willing to just "be open." It comes back to nakedness.
Can we sit naked enough that we begin to empathize with
how the dying person emotionally feels?

The only way to answer this question is to try it
for yourself and see.

If the dying person is a mother with cancer, try to
absorb by osmosis her feelings about herself. The fear of
leaving her children behind. The feeling of no longer being
sexually attractive to her husband.

For a person dying with AIDS, there may be a

tremendous shame from society. What's it like to feel ostra-
cized from perhaps your family and even your friends (who
are scared to look into your mirror of dying)?

Of course, these are generalities. With each particular person there are many specific feelings to be touched
and shared. Some painful, some joyous. You can begin
subtly. In fact, it is advisable to do so. Watch yourself and
your emotional limits. Sitting with someone who is dying
may not be the place to become swept away in empathetic
grief—but then again, it may. There are no rules here other
than to try to maintain an honest awareness of your inner
process. Also, it helps to try to relax as much as you can.
As a dear friend of mine says, "When sitting with someone
who's dying, relax and be; it's just like when I'm holding
a newborn baby, relax and be."

Connecting Beyond the Costume

Mother Teresa of Calcutta is renowned for her charity of
good works, but these deeds pale in comparison to her
charity of vision. Mother is not only a social worker, but
a spiritual advisor to those thousands of women and men
who have come to her and dedicated their lives to finding
God through the "method" of spiritual awakening she
teaches. A daily reminder of hers to her workers is that,
though our occupation is to care for the poor, our "true
vocation" is to see Jesus in the face of everyone, poor and
rich alike. She teaches a method of looking to see the face
of Christ before us everywhere. This involves a practice of
seeing beyond someone's costume of worldly self and into
the reality of holy Self. It is Mother's understanding that
we should strive to see the Light of Christ in our fellow

human being even when he doesn't see this Light in himself. (This is modeled, by the way, on Jesus, whom we spoke of earlier as being able to see all of us, saint and sinner alike, as equally loved children of God.) From a perspective of spiritual practice, the point of this type of inner work is that, as we touch upon the One Christed Self in others, we recognize that universal holiness within ourselves as well.

One way to do this is to try to literally see the Beloved within the person who's dying. We can even go as far as to personify that Beloved as Jesus of Nazareth or the Buddha. It's as if the Beloved has taken on temporary costume in order to share with us the grace of his dying. But a common problem with this method is that a forced "seeing" often encourages us to actively deny the dying person's worldly pain and process. If we remain literal to this mode of seeing, we may not be able to empathize or be fully present. We may also miss our own lessons, because we're so busy focusing beyond the surface of the mirror that we can't see what's being reflected in it. In short, it's easy to deceive ourselves with this method. In lifting us above our pain, this method can also lift us beyond our true lessons of growth. So we must be extremely conscious of our intentions when doing this kind of practice.

I once counseled a hospital volunteer who had made this practice the cornerstone of her conscious-dying work. As she would enter the room of someone who was dying, her heart and mind would soar in ecstasy, being engulfed by "the presence of Jesus." For her, the dying person was a personal manifestation of Jesus, and so each moment was precious. This gave her an immense sense of loving kindness, and her presence did seem healing to many of the people she visited. The dilemma she kept encountering, however, was that she couldn't balance the "un-Jesus-like" fears of her patients with her own feelings of the Beloved's presence. She coped by trying to ignore the patient's personality, which was angry or fearful—the result being that she wasn't truly present with her patients. Through this practice she had returned, through the backdoor, into the cure-centered approach; in this case, the cure was seeing Jesus instead of pain, suffering, and dying.

My advice to her was to stop trying to see Jesus and instead see (and then *feel*) the suffering and dying of Mrs. Smith. The way to the Beloved is not by denying the body/personality, but by loving and honoring "what is"— and honestly working with our own fears of this body's dying. The Beloved will show itself to us *if we're open*. Learning to remain open is the key. This is why I prefer to think of this practice as "connecting" beyond the costume, as opposed to "seeing" beyond it. When we emphasize seeing, we are speaking in terms of focus, which is a conscious choice, a mental decision. And usually we can't focus on two things at once. Focus is mostly either/or, whereas "connection" implies something a bit more elusive, even tactile. Connection is something we feel, something that doesn't necessarily have an image or picture attached. Connection doesn't imply either/or. We can be both connected and not. Think of it, we can connect emotionally to someone without connecting physically, and vice versa. If we open ourselves to connecting with the Beloved within a person who is dying, we can also allow the space for that person to be Mrs. Smith too. We are not seeing a being (like Jesus) other than Mrs. Smith; we are connecting to, touching, the part of Mrs. Smith herself *that is* the Beloved. Also, what part of us connects? We are on much more figurative ground here. It is not so literal as "seeing Jesus" with our eyes and mind. It is connecting within the elusive ground of heart and soul. From here we can open to accept the paradox and Divine Mystery that *both* the Beloved and the fearful human mind are present in this very person before us. From here we can look at the whole mirror, not just the reflections we've pre-scripted.

Also, from here, we can open to accept that both the Beloved and fearful human mind are present within ourselves as well.

Pain, Paradox, and Grace

There is a paradox found in the pain of dying. Anyone who's spent much time with the dying and used that time to work on their own spiritual growth has experienced this. Sometimes the pain seems plainly cruel and horrendous. But there are also times that one's pain seems to be clearly serving a greater purpose in the dying/healing process. From a spiritual point of view, it is possible to see how pain is working to awaken the dying person, and to awaken those around that person who are willing to empathize. The intense pain is wearing away the superfluous attachments, the clinging to the world, and polishing the rough stone into a clear diamond.

Those who have worked with the dying are familiar with a certain scenario. The form is always a bit different, but the essence, the heart, is the same. It could happen something like this: There is grandma, tired, pumped full of medications, soon to die of cancer. And maybe grandma is not particularly liked by all the family. Perhaps she has had a hard life these last years and is bitter and resentful. A relative has taken it upon himself to care for grandma while she dies. He puts up with her abusive personality because no one else will. Her heart seems filled with fear, anger, and judgment. Hardly anyone escapes her criticism.

Or, maybe it's this way: There is grandma who is very much loved by everyone. She's "Granny" after all; they all know her so well, remember so many Christmas mornings at her house. The family would know her particular smile anywhere because grandma has a particular smile for her particular grandkids. You knew grandma loved you, and you were special to grandma, one of her special children. Everyone loves grandma and is saddened that she is about to die.

Either way, it doesn't matter.

Because it happens to all types of grandmas, and grandpas and children and grandchildren. What happens is a "hatching." The shell of the ego cracks much like the shell of an egg. Whether it's the intense and prolonged pain, whether it's the clarity of what's truly important in the last few days, or hours, or whether it's a little of both— it doesn't matter. But those who've worked extensively with the dying know what I mean. The shell of grandma's ego-identity cracks, and what emerges seems like someone else entirely.

Suddenly grandma's not the same old grandma anymore. She doesn't *see* her family in the same way she did before. Old wounds and grievances are healed. Or the special love she once held only toward certain members of the family is now extended to everyone: doctors, nurses, everyone, even former "black sheep" family members. This shift can be frightening to those who still want to see the old grandma. The truth is, "grandma" has gone. Her shell of self-identity has been laid aside. Quite often this new awareness is dismissed as "drug induced" from pain medication. But if you spend time with her, you'll see that she really has changed. The spiritual traveler we believed for so long to be "grandma" is, in actuality, awakening into her larger reality—the sacred self. Suddenly this being called "grandma" is beholding the world through the mind and eyes of a Christed being. And when this process begins in earnest, "grandma" falls away like the broken shell of an egg during hatching. If you are honored to be present at such a hatching, recognize it for the miracle it is. Be thankful to be in the presence of such an emerging being. Spend as much time with her as you can.

In the hospital, I noticed that upon this emergence of sacred self, either the body goes on to be laid aside with the ego shell or, sometimes, the body undergoes a form of unexpected physical healing. If the body heals and remains here a while longer, it is not at all certain that the freshness of this awakening will remain intact. Quite often, the clarity of this profound awakening will lessen in time. But not always . . .

The paradox for those of us trying to be alive in the presence of someone who is dying is stark: the pain is an integral part of Grandma's awakening process, yet we certainly couldn't give her that pain (or even wish it upon her). We, with our emotional hearts, want to remove every bit of that pain and suffering. But another part of us recognizes quite clearly that, in this situation, the pain is grace.

This is not a statement to be adopted flippantly: *the pain is grace.* It takes a leap in consciousness to truly come to know this. Like all other matters of growth along the journey, we may understand it intellectually, but ultimately it is a lesson of the heart. To really know that pain is grace, we must begin to see with a more spacious vision. This is part of the reason why we don't say to someone who is suffering, "Don't complain, it's really grace." To authentically come to this understanding, this channel of perception, takes time and experience. It takes a softening to life. As we practice living our dying and begin to see how suffering is grace from one perspective, we also come to appreciate that not everyone is at the place in their journey where they're ready to join us in our more spacious perspective. Often, what a dying person wants is straightforward: compassion and empathy for that person's plight, right here in the dirty grit of hell on earth. It is on these occasions that our experiential realization of "suffering is grace" can allow us, paradoxically, to enter even deeper into another's pain. "Suffering is grace" is not a doctrine to be preached, but a personal experience to be felt for oneself.

Once we start to awaken spiritually, we take another look at pain and suffering—Grandma's and our own—and start to perceive both as a vehicle to awakening. Yet the paradox remains: *we still feel the pain. Perceiving pain as grace doesn't stop us from feeling the hurt or from wanting the pain to end. The way to the sacred is filled with paradox.*

Softening and Grieving

To be alive with someone who is dying is also to be willing to grieve, now, before they die. If we cannot open to grief, we cannot open to love or compassion either. As Stephen Levine puts it, "It's hard to kiss someone when you have a stiff upper lip." Yet how can we grieve, how can we open to that almost unbearable pain when it arises within us? We may feel that if we open and let the floodgates down, we'll be swept away in the resulting deluge. This may be so, but not always. How can we cultivate the courage and compassion of opening?

Instead of "opening and closing," consider the image of "softening and hardening." When we encounter feelings of grief, usually our response is to harden ourselves, harden the armor around our hearts. It is a mode of self-protection and survival: the stiff upper lip, the heart hardened to pain and suffering. This understanding of how we harden comes from the conscious-dying work of Stephen and Ondrea Levine. It has been immensely valuable to me in my own process, not just because it's true, but because there exists a simple, profound practice to break through this hardening, which is called "softening the belly." In their book on conscious relationships, *Embracing the Beloved*, Stephen and Ondrea Levine write:

> This armoring of the heart is recognizable as a hardness in the belly. The belly has become rigid with holding. It is a reflection in the body of the imprisonment of the mind. . . . This hardness reminds us to soften, to let go into healing. Soft belly is open belly, is direct access to the heart.
>
> When we begin to soften the belly, we discover we

have room for it all. . . . Room to heal. Room even to die with an unencumbered heart.

Room to grieve openly and live our dying now, not later. The practice of softening the belly when we feel fear is a key for awakening into a more conscious life. It is a spiritual advisor that never lies: if the belly is hard, it is time to soften, soften, soften.

One of the primary benefits of this practice is its immediacy. It can be done anywhere at any time. Like other practices, softening the belly becomes easier the more we do it. This softening certainly need not be reserved for special, high-pressure situations. In fact, as we become more aware of ourselves and our bodies, we come to realize that the belly lives in an almost constant state of tightness. Over the years, most of us have stored up layers and layers of armoring around our hearts, which are also layers of tight-ness in our bellies. There is much softening to be done. It is a constant practice, and the most powerful means I know to soften into our grief and true emotional heart. (For a detailed guided mediation to this practice, you may wish to see the writings by Stephen Levine in the "Suggestions for Further Reading" at the end of this book.)

Certain spiritual traditions advise us not to grieve too long for a person who has died. The implication is that, if we continue to think of the deceased in our consciousness, we somehow keep his or her soul from continuing on to com-plete its journey. I'm suspicious of that. I feel a bit like

C. S. Lewis when he doubted the validity of the statement, "At least the person who's died is no longer in great pain." He asked, how do we know that? How do we know that the deceased person doesn't miss us as much as we miss them? How do we really know that just because someone no longer has a physical body, she is released from emotional pain too? It's a good question. Likewise, I'm suspicious of teachings that encourage us to hurriedly curtail our grieving for the supposed good of the person who has died. How do we know? If our beloved has not died but, say, has been separated from us forever by geography, would her life on the other side of the world be any less full or complete because we took our own sweet time in grieving her loss? It seems to me that to hurry up and "get over" our grief (to deny and bury it) would do little to aid the emotional and spiritual growth of the person who has died. Rather, it would more likely bypass some authentic work within *our own process* that we'll have to return to sooner or later.

Part of the theological reasoning behind this "hurry up and get over your grief so the dearly departed can travel on" is that we are all interconnected. The theory is that, since those who have died are interconnected with us, our "holding on" to them in the form of grief will likewise "hold" them from continuing their journey onward after this life. But this presupposes that they are still, after laying aside the human body, connected in an individually human way. I think our interconnection with each other and all things on a universal spirit level does not follow so linear a rule. Wouldn't our true interconnection be of a far greater magnitude than what we can conceptually understand? We are talking about nothing less than God, here, aren't we?

I believe the universe and God are far too vast, and our brother's soul far too spacious, to be held hostage to your or my individual grief process. My advice is, "Please grieve!" Grieve as long as you need to. And if one day you feel you're stuck in grief and not moving forward, seek help. But do so out of an intention for *your own* growth and development, not out of guilt that you are somehow delaying the process of someone who has died.

The Five Stages of Dying (and Living):
  Re-Visioning Our Formulas
With the publication of *On Death and Dying* in 1970, Elisabeth Kübler-Ross changed the way we looked at the dying process. While working with terminally ill patients, she identified common states of mind and, from this, formulated five generalized "stages" that the dying process usually elicited in the patient: denial, anger, bargaining, depression, and acceptance. For those healthcare workers who served the dying, the five stages began providing a structure by which to understand and comprehend the dying person's experience. It was a powerful tool in bringing down our walls around death. Yet these stages soon became popularized as a concrete, nonwavering model. It is this concretization and formulaic thinking that needs to be re-visioned. Though the five stages have given us a much needed context, we also need to be aware of the inherent traps and illusions of any context we turn into a formula.

For example, I've seen well-meaning healthcare workers and family members use these stages as merely another wall to distance themselves from the mirror dying provides. It's tempting to hide within our intellectual concepts and ideas. "Oh, she's in the anger stage, now," or "He's moving from depression to acceptance." How quickly we seek to make solid and fixed the moment-to-moment flux of life's experience. This is not to say we should dismiss the five stages (or emotional states) of dying—to the contrary. These stages can be more fully understood for how they truly operate as changing states of mind, but they can't be dismissed. They exist. They are real. Every person alive has experienced denial, anger, bargaining, depression, and acceptance; these are the feelings of loss—*any loss*, not only the loss from approaching physical death. In this way, these states are the feelings we encounter almost daily in living our dying. They most certainly need to be recognized and acknowledged. So often we think, "If I just ignore my anger or depression, it'll go away." Or we take a pill, claiming, "Time heals all." The lesson of living our dying is that we must go deeper into our fears and issues. Why not look upon these five stages of dying as states of living our dying? When we notice ourselves (or someone who's dying) working through a state of denial, we can respect and honor the experience for what it is: a moment of a larger journey into wholeness. Of course, we can encourage movement in someone's process if we feel that's appropriate. The key is for us not to be attached to where that movement goes.

From a literalist "stage by stage" point of view, the dying person's state of mind must progress linearly from denial (stage 1) to anger (stage 2); but in actual experience, the mind may move moment to moment, from denial to acceptance and then to bargaining—or whatever—on and on. If we are busy insisting that the mind adhere to a pre-scripted linear model, we will miss what is truly happening.

We will miss being alive with the dying person (and with ourselves and everyone else, as well). The primary issue evoked by the "stage by stage" or, what I like to call the "up the ladder" model, is the age-old issue of control. For many of us, when we learned about these five common states of mind, we thought we'd found a new answer. We thought: "Here's the key, and I can use it to control and manipulate the process—the dying person's and my own. With this, I can lessen the pain." Used as a means of controlling the dying process, the five stages can become a way to avoid growth and healing instead of furthering it. Again, this is not to say that the five basic emotional states are erroneous or unhelpful. The problem is our formulaic "up the ladder" approach. In reality, no journey of the heart is so nicely linear. As we noted earlier, the journey is more like alphabet soup than the alphabet song.

To talk about the stages in a larger context, the context of loss itself, we can broaden our view to include our entire life journey. How we view our life process is also how we view our dying process. Instead of focusing on the different stages or emotional states themselves, let's look at the overall movement, the model or type of structure we see beneath life's journey.

Whether we are consciously aware of it nor not, each of us maintains a conceptual model for how we see and understand our journey. As pointed out, a literalist interpretation of the five stages seems to suggest the "up the ladder" model. The ladder is a well-known symbol for progression through life: our educational system, our military, even our religious hierarchies are based upon a graduated, step-by-step progression. According to this model, as we climb the rungs of a ladder, so do we climb the path of growth, healing, and progress. Some people are ahead of us on life's ladder, others behind. The journey is viewed as rung by rung, following an upward progression. Yet, as we can see in many dying scenarios, this model often leads us to an intellectual certainty that can be used to separate us from healing, a detour away from experience and into intellectual bypasses. On the other hand, however, there do seem to be common steps along the journey that most of us share. As a tool of comparison, the ladder model can be a convenient way to discuss the shared aspects of life's journey. But convenience is not necessarily truth. In my own experience, I eventually found the ladder to be too constricting an image. As I continued working with my own living and dying issues, I began to notice another way of visualizing my life's journey. This image seemed more accurate and truthful to my life's experiential reality— the circle.

The circle is one of the oldest symbols we know, a symbol of perfection and wholeness. I believe the circle helps us share a broader perspective. Try considering your life's journey, its experiences and moments, as points or places along the circumference of a circle. In the historical fact of your journey, each point, or stage, does indeed contribute to the next, like a ladder. But since these points are along a circle, none is truly above or below the next. There is no actual upward progression along a circle; there is only the coming around. As an overriding metaphor, the circle also helps us avoid too much intellectualized self-evaluation regarding "where we are" along the journey's way. (The ego mind is quite content to study and analyze its own awakening process, for in doing so it maintains its own separate selfness through reflection and analysis.) Within the circle model our concern is not with progressing up the hierarchy. Our primary obligation is to be forthright and honest about opening into what's directly before us. The circle directs us back to the present moment. And, of course, the most striking attribute of the circle is that—in truth—it takes us no place. Ours is a journey without distance. The question is never one of place, of *where* we travelers believe ourselves to be. Ultimately, the question is one of *who* we travelers believe ourselves to be: a physical and psychological body, or a fellow soul-traveler, or at one with the Christed Self, and so forth. The circle directs us back to this ultimate question of identity, of "Who am I?"

Realizing that denial, anger, bargaining, depression, and acceptance are experiential points along a circle, we can allow others and ourselves the spaciousness to honestly feel the emotional process of spiritually awakening. We don't assume we know what's best, what "next" emotional state is proper for someone in order to grow and heal. We recognize that often a pre-scripted formula forces us to narrow our view so tightly that we miss the greater, natural movement occurring. If we are determined only to see what is acknowledged on our pre-scripted ladder, we can't see the mirror's larger reflection. So we return to the notion of a circle and lay down our linear models of certainty. We open to the unknown, to our own fears, and openly look into what the living mirror is showing us.

This is the journey. This is the immense heart of the work Elisabeth Kübler-Ross began almost thirty years ago. These states of mind are keys to tolerance and openness.

They were not intended to lock us into a forever-fixed pattern, but to unlock our blinding fears. We've come a long way since. Part of our own healing is learning how to re-vision our previous ways of looking at the world, ourselves, and each other. It is the ongoing work of taking another look, softening the belly, and letting the mirror openly reflect its truth.

Other-Referencing and Burnout

We look into a mirror in order to see ourselves; likewise, we endeavor to be alive with someone who's dying in order to heal ourselves. A chaplain who worked with terminal cancer patients once told me, "As far as I'm concerned, everything I do here at the hospital, every patient I see, is ultimately for my own healing. What I do is not about healing them or helping them find God in the middle of all this pain. It's about me finding God, coming to know myself in a richer way. So what I do here is about me healing me. It's only when I forget this that I get into real trouble."

This is perhaps the most difficult—and basic—lesson for us to remember: our work is about our own personal healing process, and no one else's. This is difficult because, on a very practical level, it seems blatantly untrue. Daily we can experience the miracle that our work seems to be about some greater, even communal healing and movement. As no one is an island, no one's healing is wholly singular. Without a doubt, the synchronistic grace of healing's power affects us all. Yet, as many of us have also realized, we can easily "get into real trouble" when we lose focus of our own personal process. That's why I've found it is best to keep this almost black-and-white doctrine of "It's about *my* healing" in the forefront of consciousness. Even though it is not wholly accurate in the larger scheme of things, this focus is still the best concept I know of in which to ground myself. Why?

To begin with, this view helps avoid the temptation of being too "other-referenced" and reminds me to concentrate on the authentic inquiry of "self-reference." After all, it is my journey I'm traveling, my life I'm exploring, not another's. It keeps me, in a way, honest to the journey of spiritual awakening. Time and time again, when I'm called to counsel a care provider on the edge of burnout, I hear, "I've given so much, I'm drained, I just can't take it anymore." Exploring deeper, usually I find that the care provider holds a mostly other-referenced point of view toward the work. She or he is doing the work almost wholly for the "other" person's benefit. To put it another way, the dying person is the focus of all inquiry. Often there is a hidden psychological agenda—like, "If I'm good enough and give enough and am selfless enough, I'll be truly loved and appreciated (by parents, friends, God)." This is a common agenda for most of us; I speak from my own personal agenda, here. Yet, if we remain other-referenced in regard to our care work, these agendas usually remain hidden and unconscious. Overwhelmed by the process of caring for someone who's dying, we never get to the reflection of true self-inquiry. We become focused on the other's pain, and not our own. It is a powerful way to avoid confronting our own inner pain and fears, our personal doors through which we need to pass.

A friend of mine once mockingly called this intense

form of other-referencing and selfless service the "Mother Teresa Syndrome"—insinuating that it accurately models the Catholic nun's selfless giving and form of spiritual activism. My friend was right in evoking Mother Teresa as a role model for service, but for the wrong reasons. If you read Mother Teresa's writings (or talk for any length of time with one of her sisters), you'll find out that, quite bluntly, her emphasis is not on helping the dying. Instead, her primary focus is dramatically self-referenced. As mentioned earlier in this chapter, Mother's method for spiritual growth is to see the face of Christ in everyone she meets—from the Pope to the thief on the street. This is what she calls her "true vocation." The compassionate action of serving and helping the poorest of the poor and the dying is simply "my occupation," the vehicle by which she and her sisters practice seeing the face of Christ. So her spiritual program is quite self-referential. Daily the sisters confront deep questions of how their worldly walk conflicts with their spiritual talk: "Why can't I see Christ, here, in this dying man's agony?" "Why did I recoil in fear when the leper reached out to me?" "How can my God allow this immense pain and suffering I see?", and so forth. Though hundreds of thousands are served and cared for by Mother's sisters, the focus ultimately returns to the individual care provider working on her own process of experiencing Christ in everyone, her own process of spiritual deepening and awakening.

Also the practice of self-referencing is an important key for avoiding burnout. *If our work and experiences with those who are dying can be focused into "what I'm learning about myself and human nature," we can survive the burnout most care providers experience.* If we don't focus toward life in this way, we'll burn out sooner or later, probably sooner. I've worked with conscious-dying teachers who find themselves drained and depleted after each workshop they facilitate. Inevitably they see their job, as workshop leader, as providing a safe space where love and compassion abound for the participants (most of whom are facing some life-threatening disease). Their work consists of a great outpouring of their personal love and spiritual energy—and afterward they are spent. I've found myself in similar situations. I forgot that my primary focus needed to remain on my own self-inquiry, my own growth and deepening. Caught in the illusion that care was a one-way street (with me as the Great Dispenser of Love & Light), I found myself continually exhausted and feeling lost. Again, here the key is to return to the basic question of "Why?" Why am I doing this work? To be of service to others or to heal and deepen myself?

This is one of the reasons the title of this book is living *our* dying. We are not simply being with others who are dying. We, you and I, are dying ourselves. It is about you and me, personally and individually. From this space of individual responsibility we are better able to keep a wider focus on ourselves as soul-beings in a process of spiritual development and growth.

In our continual return to self-reference, we are not the youthful Narcissus longing for himself in the pool's reflection. Rather, we are the awakened Narcissus who realizes it is into depths beneath the surface reflection that we must next explore. It is a journey into this deeper reflection that ultimately leads back to a greater love and realization of self. This is not "self" as object of desire and infatuation, but a depth of sacred-self experience, awareness, and healing in the broadest sense. So if I had to choose only one image, principle, or thought for this chapter to emphasize, it would be this: finally, we must each come to understand we do this work for our own personal healing; we look into the mirror to see our own reflection, to soften to it and awaken into our own inner hearts.

The mirror awaits us. She awaits our hand extended not in judgment of how she should die or what she should feel. She asks only for our opening hand and heart. We need do nothing, say nothing. We need only sit bedside and be naked with her. It is our form of meditation, prayer, and practice. We sit again and again. Opening again, closing now, then awareness, okay, opening now. Forgiving ourselves. Having patience. Letting our process take time. It's taking time. Opening again, perhaps for a little longer now. Coming up against seemingly solid walls of fear; closing. But waiting, having the courage to go sit with her again, as she lies dying. Seeing ourselves in her eyes. Coming up to the wall again, but it's less solid now. Opening again, closing again. Letting our process take time. Having compassion for ourselves on this journey. For we know that if we sit naked with another who is dying, we may one day be able to walk naked out into the world. This is the fruit of the spiritual journey. Returning to our naked innocence. Re-visioning the world. Healing it in our innocent sight. Connecting with Christ not only in the face of the dying, but in everyone. So we sit and practice our nakedness with a dying friend, or stranger, or parent, or lover, or child. We sit and open up. As the garden returns in full bloom. We sit with living and dying alike, naked, open, and unashamed of our birthright as children of God. And look into the mirror.

Moment to Moment ... and the Moment of Death

Death tells us that we must live life now,
in the moment—that tomorrow is
illusion and never comes. It tells us that it
is not the quantity of our days, or hours,
or years that matter, but rather the quality
of the time spent. Every day is new.
Every moment is fresh.

—LEO BUSCAGLIA

I remember the first time someone asked me to assist her in dying. She was a mother in her late forties, with a wide round beautiful face that was not uncommon for the rural people of northeast Texas. Though she was on a morphine drip and not, in her own words, "in too much pain," the tumors in her had grown to such a size that they pressed against her spinal column, paralyzing her from the upper chest down. Almost every function of life had to be performed for her. She couldn't urinate or defecate for herself, or even press the buzzer to call a nurse. Her doctors didn't know how much longer she would live, perhaps another week, perhaps a bit more or a lot less. It could be a withering, slow death.

When I walked into the hospital room, her husband put his chin to his chest, shook my hand, and excused himself without looking me directly in the eyes. He left the room, glancing down to the floor. A teenage daughter was also present and though there were tears in her eyes, she was smiling. "I'll be outside," she said. "Momma wants to be alone with you."

As I moved bedside, I noticed the glow you sometimes see around those who are in the final stages of their dying process. "Hello, my name's Joseph. I'm the chaplain. The head nurse said you wanted to talk to me." The wide thick face softened more as she smiled. Her eyes glistened.

It was as if she reached out her hands and gave me a long, slow embrace, as sweet and thick and moist as those east Texas summers she had lived her whole life through. But of course only her face had moved. Everything else was still. "Yes, Honey, I wanted to see you. They told me you do other things than just regular preaching and praying."

She watched me closely. I nodded, not quite sure what she was getting at. The woman tilted her head toward the bedside table. I saw a copy of Bernie Siegel's book *Love, Medicine and Miracles*. "I've been doing the kind of things that Doctor Siegel said to do. Visualizations an' such. I think they helped some, but they didn't cure me. I'm not in too much pain right now, but sometimes it gets real bad. They don't know how much longer I've got." She smiled and closed her eyes for a moment. She seemed to float off somewhere for a few seconds but then was back, eyes shining at me. "I'd like to know if you'll help me do something?"

"Of course," I said softly. "Anything."

"Well, I'd like for you to do a visualization for me. I want you to help me go ahead an' die. Can you do that, Honey? Can you do me a visualization where I just go into God's arms an' don't come back?"

I felt my stomach grab and my breath stop. At that moment it was clear to me that everyone else in her family knew what was happening. They'd paid their last respects and had been waiting for me to arrive and do what Momma wanted. There are no words that can begin to convey how, in that moment, my heart broke at her pain, at my own pain, at the whole world's pain. Or, at how, in that same intolerably painful moment, God was also right there in all His grace and strength. And I felt a tingling of fear, but a good fear, a grounding, humbling fear—truthfully, an awe at this very moment. A sacred paradox. Her eyes shimmered, vibrant black dots of total aliveness and invitation. "Will you, Honey?"

I spoke carefully and slowly, "Yes, I can try."

She closed her eyes and the gentle smile softened as her face smoothed out into a deep, peaceful sea. "Thank you. I'm ready now. Go ahead."

At the time I was asked to do this, I had been a chaplain for maybe two weeks. I hadn't had time to prepare for such a thing—this ritual of passage. Of course I'd read conscious-dying meditations in books, but I had never actually led one. (I had led similar meditations at our Healing Circle support group, but then the point had always been to go "into the light" *and then come back.* In this visualization, there was no coming back.) I tell of my inexperience with doing this sort of care because, in doing any kind of con-scious-dying work, there is always a first time. It's important to understand that, whether our egos consciously know it or not, we are usually ready—if our hearts and intentions are in the right place. There's an old religious saying that goes, "You are never called upon to do something for God unless you're ready to do it." On a level far deeper than the conceptual, I understood that this was a great gift being offered to me. This beautiful woman, this ancient sage, was blessing me with my own initiation into faith and trust. She *knew.* And it was time for me to taste of that knowledge, as well. So she closed her eyes, snuggled back into God, and told me, "I'm ready now. Go ahead."

I did the visualization. When I finished, she was unconscious. I don't know if she ever awoke or not; she died later that night. But even if she had gone on to awaken later, or not lost consciousness during the meditation, even if she had looked up at me immediately after my finishing and said, "Honey, this visualization didn't work either; I think you're full of it," it wouldn't have mattered. Nothing could change the fact that something had died in me—and, I believe, in her. I believe that every time I've done a guided visualization to facilitate someone in completing their dying process, something has died in both of us. There is a letting go into the moment by moment by moment . . . an uncertainty of where the visualization is going, of its ending and completion. During these heightened times of awareness, I find that I'm doing this work for the One

Self—the commingled souls into a Godself—that is both me and the other person. It's a psalm praising God's love. An offering, the acceptance of an initiation rite. During a joining of such holy intentions, parts of us both die into the light and don't come back.

What died in me? In a manner, my fear died, consumed in the moment-to-moment experience of life—which we might call grace. This is a very delicate healing process and some of the most vital work we need to understand in living our dying. Metaphorically, it is an inner dying process and subsequent rebirth.

On a very literal level, this woman who was in the final stages of her dying had something I wanted. What could this have been? She had a moment-to-moment existence. She had a fearlessness about death—going "into God's arms." She had a plain, straightforward way of speaking about her pain that cut through my defenses. Perhaps the simplest way to say it is: she was as close to death as one gets in this life, and still she wasn't scared; she didn't want to run away; she wanted only to complete her living/dying process. I sensed no anxiety about her, none of the desperation that sometimes accompanies someone's wish to die before a disease progresses into its final moments. She seemed to be coming from a different level of mind entirely. And as I proceeded, I actually felt she knew on a deeper level that she was offering a gift to me, for me. She was offering to share intimately her experience of being that close to death without fear. This was the "something" she had that I wanted.

I'd come to the chaplaincy to experience and face my own fears of dying. In hindsight, I can understand that if this patient had been a man dying with AIDS, the situation may have been too fearful for me to let go into a healing. In the actual circumstance, however, it seemed as if she embraced me and held my hand every step of the way. My experience with her was an opportunity for me to move out of my intellectual-head and into my emotional-heart and experiential-body. As I said, I'd read the meditations on guiding someone to death's door before. But reading to myself was one thing; standing forth and taking the trip with someone who was willing to go "all the way" was quite another. I came up against my bodily fears, the tension, the heavy pulling in my stomach. I came up against my emotional fears. And then moved through them—guiding the visualization, following along with her. When we openly connect with someone in the final movements of the dying process, we come about as close as anyone can get to the ultimate letting go. It need not be so dramatic as facilitating someone in a guided visualization of dying. *It need only be an open, honest, and willing connection.* We open through our own fears and re-emerge on the other shore. The other shore is a moment-to-moment experience of life. With this beautiful sage I came as close to the ultimate letting go as I'd ever been. Part of me died too.

Though this particular experience was a radical step, in the whole of my experience most inner deaths have been subtle and gradual. An honest sharing of thoughts and fears with someone. A softening of the belly. A gentle tear. Or a flood of tears. A courageous joining of hearts and intentions as two people openly look into each other's eyes without speaking a word. The possibilities are endless.

In our work with living our dying, often what dies is a "protective idea" we have about ourselves and life. A protective idea of self—of defensiveness, of fear—dies and is reborn into an immediate experience of opening and spaciousness. This is what I understand as resurrection. Metaphorically, the fearfully closed and separate mind dies and ascends from the head into the heart and full body, where the mind, no longer separate but whole, is felt and known in a whole living moment of experience. No longer is our connecting to God and our fellow human beings a mere concept, but a living, breathing reality. No longer lost in thoughts of correctness and incorrectness, of self-definition and protection, we are simply open to the moment-to-moment "what is" of life before us. This is living in grace as I understand it. Moment-to-moment resurrected life.

To this day, when I visit someone who is nearing the final stages of the dying process, I still feel a resonance of the same feeling I experienced when this woman first asked me to help her die. This resonance might be described as a "little fear" tingling inside me. For me, it's located just below my navel and deep within. My visual image is of a peach seed: that hard, shriveled, hollow core at the center of a peach. It's a tightness that grips—and if I let it continue unnoticed and unacknowledged, it can grow to grip my entire body, heart, and mind. This hollow core is the secret, personal place where I do my most earnest work of letting go and softening. And when I soften and open to who I'm with, and to my self and my fears, I also feel a resonance of the safety and grace, the greater trust I later experienced with this same dying woman. I feel her embrace, the Beloved's embrace.

Yet my "little fears" still arise. Perhaps they never go away fully. Perhaps they are ultimately what makes us human. I don't know these answers. But "finding an answer" has never brought me any closer to the whole mind-body-soul integration of the moment-to-moment grace I experience when willing to go deeper into my little tight fears. I've become suspect of finding formulaic ways to explain or understand this miracle. Grace doesn't follow the linear laws of the world. It must be lived and experienced moment to moment.

The Story of Milarepa

A model for us to consider while working with our inner fears is the great Tibetan saint, Milarepa, who lived over 800 years ago. Milarepa is a good model for many reasons. He is endeared to the Tibetan people because, before he began his conscious spiritual path, he was about as far from God realization or enlightenment as is possible. In their belief system, to kill another human being almost disqualifies one from attaining any great spiritual realization in this lifetime—and Milarepa was a mass murderer! So it is fair to say Milarepa was definitely handicapped from the start. Yet, he demonstrated the almost impossible: he did in fact become enlightened within his single lifetime. He awoke despite his evil beginnings. For the Tibetans he represents hope and the idea of supreme redemption—the belief that "If poor old Milarepa could convert his wretched life to one of grace, I must certainly be able to, as well." Again, we touch upon the theme that the Christed potential is within us all—a powerful principle to keep in mind.

I mention Milarepa as a model, however, for a more specific reason. One of the stories from his life involves his meeting of the three demons. In this lore, the demons were actual beings who came to haunt the saint as he was meditating in a cave one day. We, on the other hand, can understand these creatures to be inner demons and conflicts that arose from his own mind. For us, these inner demons may represent all the inner fears, little and great, that we encounter in our daily work of living our dying. The model I find so instructive is how Milarepa deals with these arising demons.

In the story, as he sits meditating, Milarepa sees three demons appear at the mouth of his cave. These are particularly nasty, angry demons, rattling skulls, shrieking, exuding awful odors, waving bloody swords, and shouting obscenities. According to legend, as the demons enter into the calm meditative space of his cave (his consciousness), Milarepa smiles and welcomes them wholeheartedly, begging them to sit with him by the warm fire and to "take tea." The demons growl, "Aren't you horrified by our appearance?" And Milarepa replies something like, "Oh, not at all. It is at moments such as these that I am reminded to have compassion and mercy for myself. When the demons of fear, doubt, loathing, and anger appear, I am most grateful to be on the path of healing and awakening, for then I can welcome you and open my heart to you, instead of running away and hiding. So, please, come and sit. Take tea with me. You are always welcome to emerge from the darkness and sit with me by the light of the fire. For it is only here that we can take tea together."

The important images I find in this story are, of course, the opening to and welcoming of one's inner demons as they arise. But the legend also goes beyond a welcoming acceptance of our darker sides. Milarepa goes on to invite our demons to take tea with us, to join with us in intimacy by the warmth and light of the fire. I see the light of the fire as representing the illumination that comes from the often fiery circumstances that touch our lives. I am reminded of what Viktor Frankl, a survivor of Nazi concentration camps, once said: "What is to give light must endure burning." Instead of pushing our fears away from such growth-filled experiences like dying, we can invite them closer, invite them to join us beside the fire itself. Though we may in some ways be "turning up the heat," we are also increasing the potential for illumination. Likewise, if we invite our fears to join us in intimacy—to take tea with us—we can begin to understand that our fears are also living, breathing aspects of ourselves. Perhaps we may begin to honestly and compassionately say, "You're not so frightful after all. You just need to be loved and accepted. In fact, I bet you have a lot to teach me about myself. Share your heart with me, oh demon, as we sit here together and share this tea." Here we return to the care-centered approach discussed earlier, as exemplified by the Greek minotaur myth: the terrifying beast at the center of our labyrinth is also an angel.

At one point in my personal process, I thought the resonance of fear I often felt upon first entering the room of someone who was dying was something to be ashamed of. I certainly didn't invite that inner resonance to tea, let alone look up and acknowledge its presence. I tried to hide this feeling. "After this much death-and-dying work," I thought, "I should be well past this 'little' fear. If I ignore it, it'll go away." Of course none of these tactics worked. As pointed out earlier, this resonance of fear is still right here, within me today. The difference now is that I *try* to invite it to tea, to cherish its intimacy. In a manner, this resonance has become strangely comforting to me, because when I feel it I'm reminded there remains greater work to be done. It reminds me there is a resurrection to occur wherein we all sit together by the fire and share its light and warmth. The German poet Rainer Maria Rilke wrote:

> Perhaps all the dragons in our lives are princesses who are only waiting to see us act just once, with beauty and courage. Perhaps everything that frightens us is, in its deepest essence, something helpless that needs our love.

As I'm coming to spend more and more time with this inner fear, I'm coming to appreciate that it is not something that truly dies and is reborn as something else. Here, death and rebirth are metaphorical descriptions. To be more pre-cise, I believe this fear and pursuant opening are *one single* aspect of a larger healing process that cannot be separated from the greater movement. The demon is not one side of the coin, and the angel the other. They are both one whole coin, one whole movement of grace. If my fear is a figurative seed-core of a peach, we might see the peach itself, the juicy fruit that pleases and nourishes us, as always contained within the seed. We can have no peach without a seed— but also, paradoxically, no seed without a peach. Like the chicken and the egg, neither can come into being first. Each is not a separate entity, but a different aspect of one whole that cannot truthfully be divided in two. And notice that I'm back to speaking in metaphors. Once again, non-figurative language fails us as we enter that realm of experience that passeth literal understanding.

From a Nurse's Journal

A week after my friend Jeff died, fifty or so of us gathered around a lone tree in back of his house in Galisteo, New Mexico. We each took turns sprinkling Jeff's ashes into the open ground around the tree's roots. And those who wanted to say something, told their stories. It was here I heard the remarkable account of Jeff's moment of physical death as experienced by the nurse who was caring for him. I'll let it speak for itself. She read from her private journal:

I was in the bed next to him stroking his head with
*   my fingers,*
my cheek on his mouth and nose,
his breath moving the fine hairs of my cheek.

I could hear the movement of his heart with my
*   stethoscope*
and with my hand on his chest, I felt its vibrations.

His dad asked me if he was dying. I looked up into
*   the man's eyes*
and saw needful searching,
tenderness and painful courage.
I nodded my head and told him to get the others.

Then Jeff and I were alone and I closed
my eyes and gently slipped into his soul.

There I sensed lightness and anticipation.

He took only two more breaths. Then I heard
the sound of silence, his heart no longer beating.

I could follow his soul for only a few seconds more
*   and felt*
a lightness like freedom surrounding his soul.
Then euphoria.
Euphoria was all around us.
His face renewed in light and softness.

Without speaking, I said, "Fly babe fly."
Then he was gone and I was now back
lying in bed aside his body, this body
that served him so well in life.

Within seconds of his death, he was again
surrounded with the love of his family and friends.
What a way to go.

Thank you Jeff for letting me
share that intimate moment with you.

part IV

LIVING OUR DYING

*Today is a good day to die for all the things
of my life are present.*
　　　　　—CRAZY HORSE,
　　　　　　　A NATIVE AMERICAN ELDER

Relationships

'Til the first friend dies, we think ecstasy
impersonal, but then discover that he
was the cup from which we drank it, itself
as yet unknown.

—EMILY DICKINSON

When the awareness of death and dying consciously enters a relationship, the ecstasy of
true intimacy blooms brighter than we could
have ever imagined. I know of no greater way to accelerate
a deepening of intimacy within a relationship than to openly
cultivate the awareness of each other's dying.

It was only in my most recent relationship that I
first began consciously facing the fact that, most likely, my
partner would bury me one day. His immune system was
much stronger than mine. Of course, coming to openly deal
with this issue was a two-way street; we were both willing
to try to honestly include our dying within the relationship.
Still, in many ways it was easier for me. As the person
dying first, my loss seems somewhat comforted by the under-

standing that I would be embarking on a new and unknown journey in spirit. As the person remaining here in body for a time longer, my partner could expect the painful familiarity of his own illness compounded by the great loss and grief of my sudden absence from his daily life. The poet Maya Angelou writes, "I can accept the idea of my own demise, but I am unable to accept the death of anyone else. I find it impossible to let a friend or relative go into that country of no return. Disbelief becomes my close companion, and anger follows in its wake." How familiar. It is important that we work to open to the death of those we love, now, before they die—to open into our disbelief, avoidance, and anger. Don't we want to soften our hearts and remove the hidden walls between ourselves and those we love? When my partner and I first realized this, we began investigating ways in which we might begin opening to this eventual experience of loss. We began consciously talking about my death or his, and about the other's survival. It was a painful unearthing, but it created an openness and intimacy that flowed over into many other aspects of our relationship. From this ground of honesty a tender preciousness grows. Since then, it has become clear to me that our hidden fears need to be voiced to those we love. For it is when our fears remain hidden, uninvited to "take tea" beside our fire's light, that their power over us is maintained.

Another part of the reason we must consciously invite dying into our most intimate relationships has to do with the idea of purpose. We have relationships for a purpose. On surface levels, there seem to be many different reasons for our relationships: economic, psychological, cultural, reproductive. But, in truth, a deeper purpose lies at the heart of this yearning to connect and relate with others. This deeper, we might even say spiritual, purpose is succinctly expressed by this anonymous poem:

> *I sought my spirit, but my spirit I could not see;*
> *I sought my God, but my God eluded me;*
> *I sought my brother and found all three.*

Our relationships are the intimate ground upon which the soul flowers. It is within our relationships that we experience firsthand the painful losses of letting go and surrender, the aching impermanence of life. When speaking at memorial services, author Marianne Williamson often addresses the surviving loved ones directly and, acknowledging the tremendous loss and grief of the moment, says something like: "I know you feel you'll never be the same, and you're right. Out of this pain two ways are possible. You will become harder or you will become softer." This is the transformation our relationships offer to us. If we consciously invite an awareness of living our dying into our relationships now, before our physical deaths, we can begin to accept that transformation, now, as well. In conscious relationships we must come to this dilemma daily: here, we have the choice of softening or hardening our hearts to one another, moment to moment.

A nurse overseeing a large facility that specializes in care for the elderly told me bluntly, "It's the most amazing thing; hardly anyone talks about what their life has been like, or what wonderful things they've done. They only talk about what they haven't done, what they didn't get a chance to do with their husbands or wives." I've found this to be true in many situations where one partner survives the other. Of course there is sadness for what can no longer come in the future, now that a partner's beloved has died; but there is also an almost overwhelming grief (often much more profound) for what did *not* happen in the past—for opportunities lost and taken for granted. One partner cried, "I never really cuddled or snuggled with him the last few months of his life. We had no time for romance. We were just so busy fighting the disease." One can't help but wonder how different the texture of these lives might have been if living their dying had been openly and honestly cultivated throughout the relationship. Often being "busy fighting the disease" is a pseudonym for being busy avoiding the big empty spaces of dying. If we can come to realize the preciousness of life's each moment, our relationships will begin to take on a sublime intensity.

Also, it is important to understand that we have relationships with everyone and everything. These practices are not exclusive to our primary romantic relationships or life-partners. In the remainder of this chapter, I use the somewhat generic word "beloved" to represent this larger understanding of relationship. Our beloved is anyone we love: it could be a husband or wife, a lover, a child or parent, or close friend.

How can we sincerely and honestly live our own dying with someone who is not consciously aware of his or her dying? This is an important question. All day long we encounter people who are "closed" to life's mystery and haven't begun to awaken to their own dying. Earlier chapters have discussed the care-centered approach of openness, empathy, conscious speaking, eliciting, and sincere listening. These are not just attitudes and practices we adopt when sitting with the dying. These are practices for our whole lives, for us to use everyday. Likewise, many of these practices present ways to join with someone who is not consciously interested in living his or her dying. In this chapter you may use all of the following practices in a "solo" form, whereby your beloved is not consciously aware of your work. This is often the case when parents or children are involved. As you do the inner work on yourself, however, be open for a newfound softening to appear in those around you. The work we do on softening our own hearts is often infectious.

A Basic Practice: The "As I Lie Dying" Letter

One of the practices described earlier in Chapter 5 was letter writing, more specifically, writing an "as I lie dying" letter. This practice involves writing a "final letter" from your imagined deathbed. For this particular exercise, you would address this letter solely to your beloved. Begin with, "Dear [your beloved's name]," and start writing. If possible, have your beloved do this practice with you, writing their own "as I lie dying" letter to you. I suggest working on this for several days. Go deep into intimacy and honesty. Set a date for you both to meet together with the finished letters. Let that time be a sacred time. Don't plan to share your letters with each other in the morning before work, or when you have a pressing engagement. Give yourself some space. You may even want to play soft instrumental music, lightly in the background. (Also, it will facilitate the work if the music is especially meaningful to both of you.) When the time to exchange your letters arrives, you might want to keep in mind the following possible suggestions:

- Instead of giving your beloved the letter you wrote, try reading it aloud to him or her. Your voice's tone and texture will deepen the meaningfulness of the experience.

- After you've finished reading aloud, ask your beloved to share his or her thoughts and feelings about what you wrote.

- When your beloved is finished sharing, you do the same, sharing your feelings about the experience. Be sure to touch upon the emotions and fears this practice elicited.

Now, reverse the roles and have your beloved read his or her letter to you, and repeat the above suggestions for sharing.

This practice is effective in opening the door to conscious dying within any relationship. After completing the process, you may want to permanently exchange letters with your beloved. Rereading your beloved's letter can provide a powerful reminder of life's impermanence and become a rich practice in its own right. Also, there is no rule that says you cannot repeat this practice as often as you both wish. And you may do this practice with the different beloveds in your life. Try it with your parents, if they are willing. Or your children. (Of course, if your beloved is not willing to participate in writing the letter, you can do this practice solo. It is up to your discretion as to whether or not you choose to actually deliver the letter.) As with all letter-writing practices, feel free to play and create.

A Practice of Hope, Without Holding On

Hope is an important part of practice. For years I denied myself hope. I thought it was spiritually incorrect. How could I truly remain "unattached" or "surrendered to God's will" if I had hope for any "worldly" thing or outcome in the future. I thought the spiritual way was renunciation of all wishes and desires for anything that was material or worldly. (And that included "hope" for living a longer life, too.) But in actuality, I *was* being materialistic—spiritually materialistic. In my mind I was collecting spiritual brownie points for my nonattachment. It took me a while to see this mistake for what it was. When I began to emerge from my fog of spiritual materialism, I soon rediscovered my naturally human need for hope.

There is a slogan I've heard in some popular spiritual circles that goes something like, "Totally committed, completely unattached." It has been used by some seekers as an affirmation to describe the way they envision living their lives. I am always somewhat suspect of these types of slogans. To begin with, they are too simplistic. To live a life of total commitment, while remaining completely nonattached (to any outcome or plan as to how that life-commitment manifests), is to live in the purest essence of enlightened mind. This affirmation is not one we can program our mind to adopt by saying it over and over again; rather, it entails a profound *undoing* of our little mind's way of thinking and perceiving. It is the spiritual work of a lifetime. In fact, I know of no one who has ever been totally committed and completely unattached all of the time. Even our spiritual giants fell off the nonattachment wagon time and again. I prefer to re-vision this idea of commitment and nonattachment, using softer images. Instead of commitment to life, consider the idea of "having hope." Instead of nonattachment to outcome, consider the act of having hope "without holding on" to that hope too firmly. But I think we deceive ourselves if we claim we're not in some way holding on to our hopes. As long as the mind remembers its hopes, there is probably some degree of holding. This is not spiritually wrong; it's honest. Since we are going to hold on to our hopes to some degree, we might ask the questions: How do we hold up without holding on?

One movement toward healing is to try to envision our holding to be with open hands. Envision that our hands hold *up* our hope from beneath. There is no grasping or clutching, no enclosure within the grip. Instead, our hands are held out openly, supporting our hope as it rests upon them. There is self-willed effort in holding up, but not selfish grasping. In this image, our hope is more like a gift being offered outwardly to the world, rather than an object captured and withheld for our own uses. Also, we must be willing to let our hopes turn into a bird and fly away before our eyes. We must let our hopes take flight from our open hand, without closing our grip in an effort to keep them. When we recognize ourselves suddenly gripping at our hopes and holding on, we remind ourselves of impermanence, of the trap and futility of holding on. And, through practice, we gradually learn to let go.

Nice images, but how do we actually do this? I have no simple answers. In one manner, every living-our-dying practice espoused in this book is aimed toward cultivating the inner spaciousness to hope without holding on, to live a life of dedication and purpose while letting the bird fly away when it's time. No simple formulas exist. It is the ongoing work of a lifetime.

There has been some rich sharing between many of my loved ones and myself as I've allowed myself to have hope again. As of this writing, several new powerful medications are on the near horizon; my t-cells have been somewhat stable over the last year; and I've not had any major opportunistic infections; also, I'm loving my life in Santa Fe. I can honestly say that a year ago neither my partner nor myself seriously planned on our having any future quantity of life together; we believed my dying process had already begun in earnest. Since that now appears not to be the case, I have enjoyed the idea of having a future beyond the next six months. And, I've gotten myself attached, and lost, and away from the present moment, at times. That's part of the journey, too. Then something happens, usually a physical limitation, and I remember, "Oh, I'm living my dying." And it becomes all the richer, or all the more painful if I'm still holding on to life being otherwise. Either way, movement continues.

Over the process, intimacy deepens as we learn to have hope, become aware of when we're holding on, and then let go. It's the basic work of conscious relationships and living our dying.

Imagining the Death of a Loved One

Though painful, this is one of the most powerful practices I've ever done. You can do this alone, or in unison with your beloved. I suggest you try it both ways if you can. The instructions are simple.

Sit quietly in a place that means "home" to both you and your beloved. It could be in your living room, at a kitchen table, or perhaps in the bedroom. Still your mind as much as possible and then imagine yourself returning home, back into this very environment, from the death of your beloved. Perhaps it is the hospital from which you return, or perhaps it is the funeral service. The key is the "returning home alone," without your beloved.

Imagining yourself to have just entered the room alone, look around at your surroundings. Notice this environment that is a creation by the two of you. Feel what it is like to be alone here, now. Feel the immense pain of missing your beloved in this place that reminds you of him or her most.

Know that this exercise can be extremely painful. The everyday mind will yell, "Why put yourself through such torture until you have to! Whatever you do, don't even think about this, let alone practice experiencing it!" But the fact is that this imagined day will eventually come in reality. If not in your own experience, in your beloved's. Try not to be swayed by the ego mind's fearful warnings. Go deep into the pain here. The rewards can be great— an opening into nothing less than our soul-self.

There is no further instruction for this meditation. It is your own. Explore its pain. Dive deep, float a while, dive deeper. Feel free to work through various themes on this topic, changing it around as you see fit. As you work with this meditation, it would be particularly helpful to read C. S. Lewis' short classic, *A Grief Observed*. And, of course, share your experiences of this meditation process with someone who is compassionate to your endeavor. This meditation takes a lot of courage. For most of us, it takes much more courage to do this meditation than to imagine our own death.

Please know that I honor you for your courage in living your dying. You are healing more than just your personal self.

chapter 9

Activism

One of the most numbing experiences in my life was standing in front of Jerry's casket, officiating at his funeral. I hadn't seen him in several years. I'd recently moved back to Texas, and had talked to him only once a few weeks before. I dreamt about him that night, and when I awoke in the morning thought I should call to see how he was getting along. Just after breakfast, before I could call him, his mother called me. "Joseph? This is Laura, Jerry's mom. Jerry passed away last night. It was peaceful." I didn't say anything for a few interminable seconds, then managed to mutter, "Oh, I'm sorry."

She continued, "I don't know if he had a chance to talk to you about it or not, but he told me just last week that he wanted you to officiate at his funeral. It meant a lot to him. He said you're the only one who knew him well enough to be real."

To be real. Right. I was going to stand up in front of a hundred of Jerry's friends and relatives in the small town of Greenville, Texas, and be real about how I felt now that Jerry was dead of AIDS.

"Of course I'll do it," I heard myself say.

On hindsight, I did—at best—an adequate job for Jerry and his family. Since the service was being held in Bible Belt rural east Texas (and not in urban Dallas), I had to be careful not to offend the gathering. So I basically fashioned the service around a traditional Protestant format, quotes from the Bible, the works. I did, however, throw in a few quotes from Jerry's own spiritual preferences, which included A *Course In Miracles* and the channeled entity Emmanuel. My favorite part was arranged by Jerry's mother: a black Gospel group sang "Amazing Grace." After the service, I rode in the passenger's seat of the hearse to the cemetery. The driver and I talked about the Dallas Cowboys' chances of making it to the Super Bowl that year.

At the cemetery I said a few more words, "dust to dust," and Jerry's casket was lowered into the moist red dirt of northeast Texas. My voice didn't crack once, not a single tear. In fact, I maintained a static slight smile throughout. It was the one direction I'd received from the surviving family: "Nothing sad, let's celebrate Jerry's moving on to a better life. He would have wanted it that way."

Earlier in the day, when I had first arrived at the funeral parlor, I had seen Jerry's mom. She ran to me, grabbing my coat sleeve. "Have you seen Jerry, yet?" she chirped. "He looks wonderful!" She said this with such enthusiasm and cheerfulness, I was momentarily lost—forgetting, imagining Jerry must be waiting in the next room, dimples flashing with a big grin on his face at the elaborate misunderstanding. A fraction of a second later I realized she was asking if I'd seen Jerry's body. When I realized this, I shook my head. "I just arrived." And I was escorted to see Jerry, tucked neatly into the open casket, with its fake white silk liner.

He looked unreal. Skin tightened to his face so that you could see the skull's outlines underneath. Bad makeup job. And his hands. They just weren't right. Nothing living held its hands that way. I think this was about the time I began smiling slightly to everything and everyone. I "numbed out," smiled, and did what I thought was my job: to cheer everyone up, to transform grief into a celebration.

A slight static smile.

There is a popular misconception many people have about activism: that it must be dramatic, somewhat anger-filled, and, at least occasionally, violent. In this misunderstanding, activism is viewed primarily as an outer posture, an external event. Yet the two great activists of our century, Gandhi and Dr. Martin Luther King, Jr., were men of a deep inner activism, living profound spiritual and prayerful lives, which they credited for being the source of their strength, courage, and fortitude. From these great examples, we can begin to expand our own ideas and concepts about activism. Let's make no mistake about it, in our culture, "living our dying" *is* an activist endeavor.

Many of us have noted a paradox seen in many activist movements: the means of activism often contradict the ideals of the movement. Peace demonstrations turn violent; civil-rights and gay-rights marches asking for toler-

ance are filled with reverse discrimination, gross generalizations, and sometimes even hatred. Of course this doesn't
mean that our causes aren't just and our activism futile. But
it does ask us to take another look at our deeper intentions. If
we really want the world around us to change, first we have
to understand—as did Gandhi and Dr. King—that we must
be willing to change *within ourselves* as well. The inescapable
truth is that we too are very much part of the unjust system
we're seeking to change. Prejudice, hatred, and human evil
also live within our hearts. True activism asks for something
much more radical than outer, social change alone; it calls
for a change in our own personal, inner intentions. True
activism begins its work inside the heart and mind. It begins
with a willingness to go deeper within, to "take tea" with
our own inner shadows.

A Grounding Practice

Our activism needs the grounding and support of a practice,
otherwise we can easily lose our balance and spin off into
anger and/or unmindful acting out. Then our activism
becomes another way of separating ourselves from one
another and from God. A grounding in the deeper sense
of life's interbeingness and sacredness is the only preparation
I know to keep our activism pure—and, ultimately, effective
and meaningful. How easily we can become the twin of
the closed heart we're seeking to open and educate. I've
met many alternative medical practitioners who, as part of
their activism, attacked and belittled traditional Western
medicines as "poisons," and the physicians practicing this
type of medicine as "heartless." The persons who say these
things are unhealed healers themselves, and usually miss

the bigger picture of patient care. Their own bigotry and prejudice close them off from the most authentically powerful form their activism could manifest: a healing presence grounded in loving compassion.

A sincere practice gives us foundation for our inner work, allowing us the much needed sense of ground to stand upon. We have a method: be it meditation, contemplative prayer, chanting, doing the rosary, reciting a mantra, traditional prayer, singing, Dervish dancing, pipe ceremonies—whatever—and our method is something we can return to again and again in preparation for our activism. Many of the practices outlined in this book will help in this grounding. I encourage you, however, to investigate other practices offered by the world's great religions, as well. Our spiritual traditions offer us teachers and fellow students who exemplify the process of awakening in action. And remember, our lessons come in all shapes and sizes. Often a teacher's inability to practice what he or she preaches is the greatest of teachings. We are all fellow travelers on this journey.

(Always test your own experience of living your dying against the philosophical or theological guidance of the teacher. A true teacher relishes such a sincere student, one who won't accept doctrine blindly. For more on this, see "Religious and Spiritual Traditions" in Chapter 3.)

Recognizing the Community

Activism makes community. People gather together in common cause and like-mindedness, and a profound power is born. This has happened in all the major activist movements of our century. Living-our-dying activism is no exception. But in our activism, the community is not so apparent.

There are conscious-dying advocates, healthcare workers who serve the dying, the survivors, the terminally ill; but merely identifying oneself in either of these categories is not the same as truly endeavoring to live your dying. I've known healthcare workers who serve the dying and do so without the slightest self-inquiry; I've experienced conscious-dying "experts" who have burnt out and are just doing their work "by the numbers" without any sincere inner work on themselves; I've been one of the terminally diagnosed who certainly didn't want to think about death, let alone consciously live his dying. There are no outward standards for our community. And, as pointed out earlier, you may be consciously seeking to live your dying and be in neither of these more obvious categories. So who's the community?

In one manner, we all are. We are all dying from the moment we're born. I think it wise to keep this somewhere in the back of our minds. When we meet individuals (most people) who are not interested in examining the dying process, it helps to remember that, whether they like it or not, they are indeed part of this process. Instead of excluding them from our community, we can work on cultivating a sense of compassion for those who are still unaware of their dying. Living our dying is not simple or easy. Most of our modern world and culture will encourage us not to do the work.

In another manner, we each need like-minded friends who can support us in our going deeper into the dying process. I've found that the basic practice of "turning toward death and dying" that was mentioned in Chapter 2 will bring us into contact with others who are endeavoring to live their own dying too. And sometimes these comrades are not so obvious: a dying person in a nursing home, an older relative who's turning introspective, a parent whose child died. We need not look for understanding only among the professionals who work with the dying. Perhaps you will notice a person on the bus who is reading this book. When you do so, consider it an invitation from the universe for you to interrupt his or her reading and introduce yourself. If they squawk, tell them it's one of the practices mentioned in the "Activism" chapter. (Though this sounds a bit tongue-in-cheek, I'm sincere.) You can likewise do the same for any of the books by Stephen Levine or Elisabeth Kübler-Ross. Take the activist initiative: introduce yourself. Of course, this is not a hard-and-fast rule. Ultimately, do what you feel guided to do from within. But you may want to take another look at any inner voice that says, "Ah, don't bother her, she's busy reading. Besides, she doesn't want to meet someone else who's interested in 'living our dying.' Let her remain safely alone with the book."

Another idea is simply to start a study group of this book or any of the others listed in the "Suggestions for Further Reading." The group format can be simple: meet for a couple of hours every week to share your insights and feelings about a chapter that everyone has previously been assigned to read. You can take turns facilitating the group, or use what the Native Americans call a "talking stick." A talking stick is simply some object that designates, "I have the floor." Whoever is holding the talking stick is the only one who speaks, period. When finished speaking, the person passes the stick to the next person around the circle. (And one can always "pass" and not speak.) Try to keep the sharing personal. Also, if someone begins to cry and grieve, avoid the tendency to quickly embrace them, to "hug away" the tears, as if saying, "Shh . . . now, don't cry like that; please don't mirror my own pain back to me." I suggest that if someone is getting into emotionally deep waters, let them swim alone for a while. Most likely they are not drowning, only splashing. Give yourself and others the space to feel. And, most important, *actively practice the practices you've learned from this book—using the "d" words, conscious listening, etc.—while you are in the group.*

If the book your group is studying contains practices that will work in groups, such as guided visualizations or writing exercises, you may wish to do them together at the meetings. Use your imagination. If your intention is not to be the "local conscious-dying expert," but simply to further your own conscious-dying process, you'll do fine. The community is around us everywhere. Continue to practice openness and softening, you'll be surprised who suddenly turns up in your life's process.

Activism's Outward Movement

As we do our inner work, naturally we feel called upon to do outer works as well. Like most aspects of the journey, the line separating inner and outer begins to blur in time. For example, using the "d" words instead of euphemisms is the inner work moving outward. And, conversely, as we outwardly speak the "d" words, we observe and notice our inner reactions (a movement back within). Again, the outside-inside distinction becomes meaningless in light of our experience's interbeingness.

I remember a point in my process when I was

working on inwardly acknowledging and accepting my own dying process, and my "full blown" AIDS diagnosis. I had just started to receive Social Security Disability and was encountering feelings of personal failure and shame. (A friend told me to think of my disability as "deserve-ability," but that didn't really help then—though it is true.) One of the practices I began during this time was to be honest about my "job." Often someone asks, "What do you do for a living?" Until receiving disability, I'd always responded that I wrote and lectured on spiritual awakening and life-threatening illness. Though I was still writing and occasionally lecturing, in order to honestly integrate and accept my health's decline and dying pro-cess, I knew I had to be more up front about how I managed to pay the rent and bills. (Because certainly my writing and lecturing were no longer bringing in enough money to cover living expenses.) So eventually when someone would ask me what I did for a living, I'd answer: "I have AIDS and I'm disabled." The responses that were mirrored back to me were instructive.

Often someone's reply would be, "You don't look sick." At first I answered, "Thank you," as if my having avoided any serious opportunistic infection was a feat of personal honor. Then I began to realize this was a veiled separation, perhaps even an attack upon those who did "look" sick. And what was going to happen when I, too, looked sick—would I feel ashamed of that natural progression? I understood that the "you don't look sick" response was usually originating from deep pockets of fear and denial about dying. Obviously the person didn't mean I was undeserving of my Social Security check. Too overcome with fear to dig a little deeper into my experience, many people took the easiest route: denial. "Well, you look healthy to me."

Other times, when asked what I was writing (I like to write at coffee shops) I would say something like, "I'm a long-term survivor of AIDS and I write about conscious dying and my own experiences." Again, the responses were instructive. I'd usually be congratulated for being a long-term survivor. Nowadays, I'm not so uncomfortable with that; but as recently as a year ago, that congratulation bothered me. Again, it was as if a person with AIDS (or any other life-threatening illness) who was not a "long-term" survivor was somehow less than I. There seemed to be traces of "you must have some big secret; how special you are." I had to look deeply into myself to see if I wanted, and so elicited, that specialness (after all, I had mentioned "long term" first). For a while, I began consciously not saying "long term." Now, sometimes I say it, sometimes I don't. Mostly, I try to keep aware of my inner responses and intentions.

I'm sharing my self-questioning process to demonstrate that no outward form characterizes activist correctness. At times it may serve your inner and outer activism of living your dying to say, "I'm a survivor" of AIDS or cancer, or abuse, or whatever—but, then again, it may not. There are no steadfast rules for activist behavior. We must look within first.

Several years ago, a friend of mine was beginning graduate psychology studies at an Ivy League university whose psychology department was not known for its tolerance; it liked its graduate students to fit into a particular mold of character and appearance. My friend was not only openly gay, but dressed and acted in flamboyant and confrontational ways in order, he claimed, to bring attention to discrimination based on sexual orientation. He enjoyed the outwardly activist stance he maintained, even though it often brought him a good amount of conflict. He saw this form of activism as his personal choice, his way to teach others that "there's a bigger world out there and you'd better open your closed mind and get used to it." This served him well until he decided he wanted an internship in this conservative graduate department.

At a meeting with his graduate advisor, he told her of his desire to get an internship and student teach. He also acknowledged that his way of dressing and conduct would most likely cause conflict—which, being an activist, he was looking forward to. Her response was instructive. She said something like, "I think you need to consider that you do have the option to choose your battles here. You can continue the strategy that's served you so far: dressing against the acceptable code, wearing your sexual orientation on your sleeve, so to speak. Most likely, after a time, you will be asked to leave and, yes, that would be forcing a statement of sorts. That's one choice. But you do have others. For example, you could decide to work from within the department and conform to the outer requirements of appearance and propriety. From this space you might investigate other aspects of yourself besides your outer expression of activism. It would be a challenge for you and a challenge for your professors and students, as well. The real 'you' who is gay, and proudly so, would make himself known without the external stereotypes for anyone to scapegoat. That's another choice you have." He resisted the suggestion at first, but came to realize that perhaps she understood activism from another perspective than he. (She was, after all, the only tenured woman professor in the department; her experience with this form of activism was firsthand.) Earlier in his life process, my friend would have definitely believed that following her advice would be "selling out" his activism. Now, however, as he found himself at a different place along his life's journey, he began honestly to question the validity of his old formula. Choosing the latter strategy suggested to him, he was accepted as an intern at the Ivy League school and dressed appropriately "down," so he could teach tolerance from within. In fact, he went on to have a tremendous effect upon the faculty and students of the department as they were forced to encounter their own issues of homophobia and bigotry. His very presence of being "who he was" without any confronting external artifice was a potent form of activism.

As our inner activism becomes manifest in our lives and world, we need to understand that there are no formulas, no activist-correct stances, for us to adopt. We are each unique individual travelers, and our particular demonstration of how we live our dying will speak for itself. We may manifest our choice by quietly investigating our inner issues in therapy, or by brandishing placards noisily in a picket line. Who am I to tell you your way in any given circumstance. Here we might take to heart the Buddha's last words to his students before he died: "Be a light unto yourselves."

In this light, we can also ask what I could have done differently at Jerry's funeral. Surely, stuffing my emotions and pasting a placid smile over my heart and face wasn't activism. I've thought about this a great deal. At first, I was angry at myself for not "telling it like it is," for not using the forum to speak out about society's fear and abandonment of those who are dying. I imagined over and over again different scenarios of just what I could have done differently—of how I could have taken a more honest stand. Perhaps I could have led a guided visualization inviting everyone to imagine their own deaths. Or perhaps I could have just told stories, asked others to share stories, a deconstruction of the traditional funeral format. Or perhaps . . .

Forgetting that "denial" is a natural part of the process, I mentally beat up on myself for not having the courage or chutzpah to cut right through to a more activist perspective. In time I began to accept what had happened: I'd panicked and, in a crisis state, having to speak in front of all those mourning strangers, did the job as best I could under the circumstances. Then I began to develop some compassion for myself. I realized that the truly activist thing I could do was to have compassion for myself *now* and stop trying to second-guess what I might have done then. My present acceptance did not absolve me from a further self-inquiry, but it did free me from questioning my past outward form of expression.

The valid question for me now is: Am I cultivating the courage in my present life to more fully feel my emotions about death and dying? Had I allowed myself to truly experience my grief and sadness at Jerry's funeral, I have no doubt that the appropriate action—loving action, compassionate and healing action, truly activist action—would have become clear to me. The outward form of what I said may not have changed dramatically. Perhaps I'd have only been softer, more open, more willing to let tears fall. Or perhaps I'd have done the service wholly differently. I believe it doesn't matter. What matters is my inner intention of openness and willingness to be fully present, fully alive to the moment, pain and all. The activism naturally arises from that kind of present grounding.

Last week, at our writing group, Joan played selections from *Different Trains* (Steve Reich, Kronos Quartet, 1988), a musical piece combining string quartet, recorded sounds of old locomotives of the 1930s and 1940s, with taped recollections of passengers and a Pullman porter who traveled the New York–Los Angeles line during that era. The work then juxtaposed this particularly American oral history with the voices of European Holocaust survivors describing their own experiences of an altogether different train ride—that long ride to the Nazi death camps. It was a powerful and disturbing piece, not soothing, but cacophonous, clanking, and intrusive. As we listened, Joan asked us to write about our own train ride. "What train are you on?" she asked. "Now write for ten minutes. Go . . ."

A train towards, headlong towards death. It's not true when someone says, "Aren't we all dying? We're dying from the moment we're born, after all. . . . So we're all terminal here." No, it's not true, that statement. Though correct in intellectual fact, most of us don't know "I'm dying" in our hearts. In our hearts and emotional lives, we certainly don't. I didn't. I'm just beginning to learn "I'm dying" now. And I still forget. If I'm on a train, it's a train called "The Dying Express." Which is also "The Living Express." If I'm an activist about anything, it's about living our dying.

We run from dying. We separate it off. It's over there. In the hospital. In the hospice. In the old-folks home. Shh . . . don't tell the children. Lower your voice. Keep it in the closet. Whatever you do, don't invite "it" in. So my train is to invite our dying—yours and mine—back into the daily marrow of our lives. I am dying now. Look at me. I am dying now.

I am dying now. I am dying now. I am dying now. The rhythmic choog-a-choog-a-choog-a-choog-a-choog of the journey, the wheels along the track. I-am-dying-now. I-am-dying-now. Living-now. Dying-now. Choog-a-choog-a-choog. Living-now. Dying-now. One-process-now. One-moment-now. I-am-living-now-dying-now-living-now-my-dying-now.

The train whistle blows, screeching what no one wants to hear. We fear it. I fear it too sometimes. But we're on the train regardless. We can't get off. I can't get off.

So I'm an activist and I'm living my dying. (Or is that not putting it in true activist language. Okay, yea, I'm just dying now.) I'm dying now. Be with that truth. Open. Scream. Rage. Accept. Whatever. But be with it, authentically be with that! I'm dying now.

If we're political activists, our train is often to deny this dying. After all, the dead can't vote. (Or can they?) As healers, we deny our dying as "failure." As a community, we deny our dying in order to "give hope." Oh, we say, our HIV-positive status is not a wake-up call to dying, just a change in lifestyle. Don't panic. It's not such a big deal. Deny your fear, don't open that door! You'll fall over the precipice, into the abyss! Don't open that door! We pretend that we can live the same old, slightly modified, life . . . with our same old, slightly modified, goals and dreams. We pretend. We with cancer, we in old age, we with AIDS, with all kinds of diseases, conditions, addictions, and ailments—we pretend. It's just a "change in life-style." An "adjustment." I wonder what would happen if all of us who are diagnosed in some way, and all of us who know someone who's diagnosed, or who love someone who's diagnosed—all of us—suddenly decided to soften our hearts and open our minds courageously to "I'm-dying-now, I'm-dying-now"? How would that change our world? How?—if we let its truth enter our guts and lived with it for a while? What would our world be like if you and I and everyone embraced I'm-dying-now?

Yes, a new form of activism. Awakening to our dying. It's a train of different priorities. It begins right here, right now. Why not awaken to the ride?

I'm-dying-now. I'm-dying-now. Living-now. Dying-now. Living-now. Dying-now. Choog-a-choog-a-choog. One-process-now. One-moment-now. I-am-living-now-my-dying-now.

Now-living-now-my-dying-now.

Intimacy with All Things

To be enlightened is to be intimate with all things.

—DOGEN

L ast night, while brushing my teeth, I noticed the spot on my lower lip. It was a familiar spot in a familiar place: a fever blister, herpes. I have another on the back of my neck, just at the hair line. Because of my lowered immunity, if I don't take daily medication as a prophylaxis, these blisters would never go away. As it is now, they only flare up every few months or so. Standing there, looking in the mirror at this scarlet letter on my lip, I remembered, "Oh yes, I have AIDS. I'm dying today." It wasn't a maudlin remembrance. It was matter of fact, and then it became . . . comforting. I felt suddenly reconnected to a higher truth about myself and life. In this moment of noticing the herpes on my lip, what was comforting wasn't the fact of my disease, but the inner resonance that arose from remembering my own impermanence. As I lay in bed later that night, feeling the tingling beginnings of the blister, my heart opened to the moment-to-moment aware-ness of my daily life as it is. "Dying now," I thought, dipping down a bit deeper into life's mystery. Dying now. What a journey this is—an hour before, I'd been busily swept away in cleaning the dinner's dishes and getting the house "in order." Now, my mind was so still I felt a tender awe at my own life's preciousness. The cool bed sheets, the tingling in my toes, the heaviness of the blanket, the street lamp's light filtering through makeshift curtains—all of this was so precious, so miraculous, yet simple and ordinary. Every moment was delicate. And I knew no greater mystery ever existed than this, this exact moment of my life.

Of course, by the next morning I'd forgotten the preciousness: running late for an appointment, with wet hair in the cold mountain wind, it was me against the world, time and traffic—until I caught a glimpse of my lip in the car's rearview mirror and, again, remembered. I tell of this to prevent any misunderstanding that I might be somehow "above" the seasons of the human heart and mind. I'm not. It's human to forget. And it's also human to remember. One whole coin, remember. Divinity and humanity—the preciousness is paradoxically both.

I know of no greater way to help myself recall the pre-ciousness of life than to remember "I'm dying today." In the remembering of, the feeling of, "dying now," our every-day world reveals itself to be quite precious indeed. As we look closer at the larger context of this preciousness, another word comes to mind—intimacy. In the thirteenth century,

Zen master Dogen realized this when he declared, "To be enlightened is to be intimate with all things." We feel a deep intimacy with all things, people, places, events, with all of life during these times of inner resonance.

Growing Pains

Another paradox of the journey is that, often, our sense of grief becomes more intense as we continue to awaken. The more our heart opens, the more intense is our grief when it closes. And make no mistake about it, our hearts will continue to close again and again. There is no such thing as a static open heart, except in the ego's fiction. Life breathes. In and out, opening and closing. Our subtle work is to allow the heart its space, and that includes the space to be closed. This is the delicate paradox of opening to our closing, softening to our hardening. How easily we can slip into a formula of "open is good" and "closed is bad." How easily we choose painless comfort once again, over painful growth.

No way exists to avoid our spiritual and emotional growing pains. Why not make room for the heart to ache? Why not do as Milarepa did, invite the closure and hurt to take tea with us—not in a manipulative attempt to change the pain, but simply to let it be, to give it more space. In the Bible, the book of *Ecclesiastes* says, "There is a time for everything, and a season for all things under heaven." This is no less true with the heart. There is a season to open and a season to close. A season for everything, even, as the scripture says, "a time to be born and a time to die."

As we do the spiritual and emotional work of living our dying, the intellectual understanding that "everything dies" moves into the heart-body experience of "*all this* is dying before me now." The intellectual recognition of a crack in our "I'll live forever" egg, becomes a feeling—a resonance within. From this experiential awakening we can come to understand that nothing in life is permanent, the only constant being change itself. As we work with this, we watch our own bizarre attempts to build some kind of permanence. It spans the breadth of the dramatic, such as denying a terminal diagnosis, to the mundane, such as believing that we must keep the kitchen counters spotlessly clean. Each is a way of denying the ever-changing reality of life, and so denying the great ongoing dying process of life. It is in becoming conscious of this greater dying that we begin to see our attempts at maintaining the illusion of permanence. We begin to notice how we have illusions of permanence in all aspects of our lives: relationships, jobs, living circumstances, and especially our bodies (such as keeping a certain weight or hair color). We recognize how attached we are to controlling and restricting change— how we want to avoid pain at all costs, which is to avoid change. In one manner, all this attempted control over life's everyday experience points to a similar attempt to control something greater: our own dying. The little attachments we have as to how daily life "should be" point to our greater attachment of not letting go into our own physical deaths. From our old controlling perspective, death was the ultimate failure of gamesmanship—the game is over, we lost.

As this misunderstanding of seeking comfort and control begins to sink into our hearts, we also begin to internalize a powerful truth: our dying reminds us that life—

even everyday life—is bigger than our gamesmanship allows. No matter how hard we pray, plan, plead, or practice getting everything "just right," it still doesn't matter. The game is ultimately, and even immediately, out of our control. Within this realization, we can begin to sincerely ask, "What's the game really about, anyway?" At this point we've taken another look and realized there's a greater mystery afoot.

Everything dies. What an understanding to bring into our daily, emotional hearts! What an understanding to feel! In it we find a kind of liberation. We are liberated from the old myth of control and "getting it right." And our liberation offers no new answers or solutions. Liberation offers the spaciousness of no-answer, no-solution. We can find no "plan" to win the game. Winning is revealed as another illusion. And from here we begin to lose sight of a game altogether.

If we have no game, what do we have?

We have the moment, the opening or closing of our hearts, the connection or lack of connection. Our realization is that progress is not found through winning, but through becoming more and more intimate with life—intimate with ourselves and others, with our world, moment to moment.

Becoming intimate with all things is also getting close to our growing pains, our heart closings and seasons of fear. We want intimacy with all things because, at this point in our journey, we realize there is no other true way to live. And, yes, we get sidetracked. We forget for a while. Then we remember and come back to intimacy. We see a fever blister on our lips or our child coughing in pain, or feel a lump in our breasts or a profound fatigue in our bones—somehow we notice and remember "dying now" and, *if we've done the emotional and spiritual work*, we may begin to cultivate the inner resonance of spaciousness that follows "dying now." Our growing pains transform into invitations of intimacy and grace.

Even to the last growing pain, our final breath, we cultivate that inner resonance of fear in one moment, and of spaciousness in the next. Fear, softening. Inner resonance, grace. Dying now, living now. Breathing now, intimate now. Living my dying now.

No Big Secret

For years I thought there must be a big secret that the sages who were intimate with dying work knew. Wasn't there a knowledge and awakening that put them "over there," separate from me and my altogether too human doubts and struggles? Of course, it wasn't only conscious-dying experts who knew the big secret. The great spiritual adepts of our history knew it too, perhaps great writers and artists, and even some great statesmen like Gandhi. In my mind, they all had been privy to a special knowledge that made them almost infallible gods. If my experience differed from what any of these "enlightened ones" said, well, I must be wrong. This was what I thought the journey was about. Finding someone else who knew, and following his rules, seeing life through his eyes. I wanted so desperately for a big secret to be hiding outside of me somewhere, a fixed goal I could discover and master. I wanted an ultimate coping mechanism that was an event, so I could do it and get it over with. But the truth is: life's a process. The Way is a process.

Awakening is an ongoing fluid happening. It never stops and is never "over and done with." The Hindu saint Ramakrishna, whose devotees claimed was perfect and completely beyond his awakening process, corrected them, noting: "No matter how high the bird flies, it can always fly higher. There is no limit to realization, because Truth is an infinite sky." As far as awakening is concerned, it seems we are all a bit like Peter Pan, we can never fully grow up. This is one of the reasons many of our spiritual teachers have emphasized the childlike qualities of awakening mind. Jesus admonished us to become as little children, dependent not upon our own egoic devices, but upon God's indwelling spirit. Zen masters speak of our cultivating "beginner's mind." *A static perfection is inanimate and dead. A living imperfection is perfectly alive and vital.*

The experts and spiritually enlightened all fall into the same old traps the beginner does. I've seen it happen time and time again. There are no gods among men. Imperfection is a perfect part of our nature. Without exception, every teacher and conscious-dying authority I've quoted in this book falls into their own traps. Not only is the light in each of us, but so too is the human ego. The difference between the great enlightened ones of our history and the rest of us is not that the enlightened have no egos. The difference is, the awakened mind is not *as* mastered by its ego as is the unawakened. In the awakened mind, the ego is a servant, a tool—much of the time, but *not all* of the time.

There is a story about Ramakrishna that so well demonstrates the truth of awakened mind. He was sitting among his devotees when lunch was brought to him. Usually his lunch was prepared and served by the most trusted yogic practitioners. After all, Ramakrishna was considered an avatar, a person born fully awakened who had incarnated not to heal his own soul, but only to help humanity. In the custom of his spiritual tradition, the avatar's food was always prepared and served according to prescribed practices of sacredness and purity. On this day, however, his food was brought to him by an attendee, a woman, he didn't recognize. Shortly her identity became known. She was the village prostitute! And, to make matters worse, she had touched the avatar's food! As the story has it, Ramakrishna and his devotees recoiled in horror. In the midst of this stir, Ramakrishna's wife entered forcefully and pointed to the prostitute. "God appeared to this woman in a vision and told her that she could end her cycle of suffering and rebirth if she were to, just once, serve an avatar his food. Here is the food that she has served. And you are an avatar. You *will* eat." At his wife's words, Ramakrishna burst into laughter and joyously began eating the food.

What happened in this story? As I read it, Ramakrishna temporarily forgot that we are each the holy child of God. He lost his awakened vision and fell victim to the ego's old rules and prejudices. Now, his devotees may claim that it would be impossible for such an enlightened being to forget—that only a lesser guru would forget. But if the story is true, he temporarily forgot. So did Jesus. There are plenty of stories in the Bible where Jesus gets angry or vengeful and says some frightfully condemning and un-Christ-like things about another child of God. (For example, Jesus cursed whole city populations to burn in hell simply because the turnouts at his lectures were less than enthusiastic.) No way around it, even Jesus forgot the reality of eternal truth at times. The key is that upon remembering, the awakened self doesn't continue to rationalize its forgetful behavior. The awakened self forgives. Ramakrishna found himself caught up in believing that the cosmic joke was real for a moment; but then he remembered it was only a joke, and that the joke was indeed on him, and so he laughed. No guilt. No justification for actions. Instead, a form of self-forgiveness and the moving on to the preciousness of moment-to-moment grace.

Our awakening is ongoing all the time. Let it be so. Don't try to solidify it, or categorize it, or define it too much; especially don't think you've got your awakening figured out. Don't try to formalize a big secret. If you do, you'll forget to laugh, too.

The big secret is there's no big secret. There is merely opening to honesty and further awareness along the way. Flying higher into the infinite sky of the sacred.

Being Alive with Yourself As You Die
The Apostle Paul wrote to the Corinthians, "I die daily." Zen master Shunryu Suzuki said, "To live in the realm of Buddha nature means to die as a small being, moment after moment." Gopal, the Hindu poet, sang "Die before dying, die living." Each of these teachers were referring to the metaphorical deaths of the egoic "little self"—a dying away of our defensiveness, fears, and closures. These metaphorical deaths prepare the seeker to remain open, soft and alive to his or her literal physical death. But they also, and primarily, prepare us to remain open and alive to our moment-to-moment life. In this way is living our dying also living our

life. Metaphorically, we die and are reborn moment to moment; this is the unattached life, the life of grace. As these great teachers saw it, dying into everyday life is truly living.

This is a true description of coming to live our lives authentically. It is what this book is about. We do these practices and try to live our dying in order to live life. Yet, sometimes a misunderstanding can arise from the above statements; sometimes we take these words to mean that if we metaphorically "die now," we are guaranteed to have an easy and trouble-free physical death later. How quickly "spiritual" death turns into something we seek in order to absolve ourselves from the pain of physical death. Listening closely, one might begin to hear the beginnings of a formula. Whenever we feel the slightest vibrations of concretizing and simplifying the awakening process into a formula, it is time to step back and take another look.

I've heard contemporary seekers misunderstand the "die before you die" teaching and remark, almost flippantly, something like: "If we awaken before we die, we'll have died before we died. Then physical death, when it comes, won't matter anyway." (In fact, I used to say something along these lines myself. It was my formula to overcome my own dying fears.) It sounds lovely, and I wish it were that simple. But let's take a closer look at this line of thinking. Here's one problem: to lock this present moment of awakening into guaranteeing a "get out of jail free" card for some future moment (when you die) falsely assumes that wakefulness is a static, forever-open state. As we've discussed already, the awakening is fluid and there are times we are more awake and times we are less. All things have their seasons, moment to moment. Another problem with this guarantee is that, in truth, the future moment of death will be "what it is" along one's individual moment-to-moment process—and not what we "think it should be." Whenever I hear formulas promising how one's death moment will be experienced, I think of what Shunryu Suzuki Roshi said to his students upon his deathbed:

> If when I die, the moment I'm dying, if I suffer that is all right, you know; that is suffering Buddha. No confusion in it. Maybe everyone will struggle because of the physical agony or spiritual agony, too. But that is all right, that is not a problem.

Maybe everyone will struggle—who knows? If we struggle, our practice is simply to remain open and honest to that struggle as it arises in the moment-to-moment experience of our lives. Even if we dedicate our lives to sharing the illumination of God's light to all we meet, we will still forget at times. Still, we are human. Still, despite all our preparations, we cannot guarantee we'll not momentarily forget during those final moments of death. In one of the Gospels, it indicates that Jesus momentarily forgot while upon the cross. He pleads to God, "Father, why have you forsaken me"—as if God has, for the moment, deserted him. Obviously, here, Jesus is not grounded in the same Christed assurance that on another occasion said, "The Father and I are One." His dedicating his life to exemplifying God's light didn't guarantee him protection from spiritual agony and doubt during his dying process.

Perhaps the true liberation, as far as approaching

the final moments of physical death, is freeing ourselves from thinking we have to find some formula to protect us from our moment-to-moment experience, whatever it may be: painful suffering and spiritual agony or quiet bliss and peacefulness. Hasn't this been our misunderstanding all along—we thought we could find a magic bypass to protect us from life's pain and uncertainty? The message our great spiritual teachers each shared with us is that we must live in the moment-to-moment grace of life as it unfolds, without attachment to guarantees. No less is true for the moment-to-moment approach of physical death. As Suzuki Roshi said about the suffering and agony that might arise during his own death, "No confusion in it . . . that is not a problem." It is not a problem because, again, it doesn't matter in the spacious wholeness of God's wide Eyes. God is not keeping track of our spiritual brownie points. "Oops, I see he doubted a moment there towards the end, too bad, directly to hell for him." Or, "Oops, a doubting thought, well that's definitely a four-legged reincarnation for her." It sounds absurd because it is.

Still, some traditions do seem to espouse the "Oops, I see he doubted, so he loses" school of theology. But if we take to heart the opening lines of the *Tao Te Ching*, "The truth that can be told of is not the Eternal Truth," we can begin to make space in our minds for the different languages and metaphors in which humankind tries to imagine the One Unimaginable Reality of God. Again, it is so easy to fall into mimicking the spiritually correct script. If the correct script is "to have faith and no doubts," Jesus himself certainly failed the test for Christianity (as did Suzuki Roshi for Buddhism, if that script is "to die without struggle"). What does this tell us?

For me, the message could not be clearer. We must learn to make the space within ourselves where we can realize the utter simplicity of truly feeling what we experience, even as we die. We touch that honesty not in self-pity or anger, but in an open acceptance of the truth of who we are in that living moment. So we return to honesty, openness.

A final thought to ponder: as you near your body's death moment, what would be the most receptive and prepared state of readiness for the mind, the soul? A theological belief that paints a pre-scripted scene of spiritual propriety, or an open, self-humbling mind that admits its inability to conceive the Divine Mystery, while valuing its own self-honesty to openly feel what it's experiencing?

I think it is better to imagine that our process is not so much to die spiritually or metaphorically (an event) before we physically die, but to try "living our dying daily." This is much harder to formulize. Living our dying is not an event like "to die." Living is fluid, ongoing. It offers no false guarantees. We cannot get hold of it. Living our dying is like the present moment. When we stop to look at it, it's already gone.

We prepare and do practices not to escape our physical death when it comes, but to be fully present, fully alive for as many of life's moments as we can. If one of those awake moments is the moment of death, how nice.

If not, it's no real problem. For the next moment, the moment *after* our physical deaths, we may remember again. As our world's great spiritual traditions tell us, life doesn't end with the body. There is another moment after. And another. And another. And another . . .

"I Was Blessed—and Could Bless"

There's an old Jewish saying that the only real gift you can give someone is to go to his funeral, because you can't honestly expect anything from him in return. In other words, it's truly a gift without attachment or conditions. It's a gift that expects no reciprocity, done purely for the respect and love of life itself. So we realize that part of the power in this kind of gift without attachments is that we are bestowing our most intimate blessings in a very pure way. Our blessing is to honor and love, expecting nothing in return.

To experience the spaciousness to bless whatever comes before us—unconditionally, without attachment or expectation of any return—is the enlightenment that is intimate with all things. It begins with becoming intimate with ourselves, with the moment-to-moment experience of our hearts, minds, and souls. To be truly intimate is to bless all we encounter. This is not done ceremonially with a pomp and circumstance that brings attention to the person who's blessing. The unattached blessing often seems so ordinary, extra-ordinary. An open face. A conscious listening without seeking any "solution." A soft belly in the presence of fear. Offering care instead of cure. Feeling empathy to another's suffering. And it occurs in the most ordinary of places—not just upon the body's deathbed.

As a poet, Yeats struggled with his art and life for years. Then at age fifty, while sitting in an ordinary London coffee shop, he experienced an awakening in which he discovered life's greatest joy is that we can bless and be blessed.

> *My fiftieth year had come and gone,*
> *I sat, a solitary man,*
> *In a crowded London shop,*
> *An open book, an empty cup*
> *On the marble tabletop.*
>
> *While on the shop and street I gazed,*
> *My body of a sudden blazed;*
> *And twenty minutes more or less*
> *It seemed, so great my happiness,*
> *That I was blessed and could bless.*

How ordinary the setting. How ordinary the outward form of the action: sitting passively in a coffee shop. An activism of the heart.

I mention this so near the end of this book in hopes of reminding us that, in living our dying and cultivating our capacity for true intimacy, we are practicing the "greater works" Jesus prophesied. Authentically living our dying is one of the greatest vows of love, healing, and selflessness one can take. In this simple act is the world blessed, and the compassionate footsteps of the Christ and Buddha felt upon the earth once again.

Beginnings
Early on in this book, you were asked to remember how life's daily texture changed just after someone important

to you died. Part of the purpose of this book is to help you experience how that texture of spaciousness, of a greater unknown mystery and sacredness everywhere, can be cultivated beyond those special times. Cultivating that sacredness in the heart of your daily life is actually what it means to live your dying. We must live our dying in life if we are to live it when we die. After all, the moment of death is still another moment in daily life. If there is one message this book has tried to illustrate it is that dying and living are not separate.

In that light, this book is a beginning, not an end. This book is not an all-encompassing manual, but a pointing finger. Continue the investigation for yourself. See the "Suggestions For Further Reading." Seek out those who have worked intimately with the dying. Seek out those nearing the end of their own dying process. Seek out your own inner teacher. Listen to everything, but embrace a teaching through testing it in relation to your own life experience. And please be willing to question everything you've read so far in this book. It's your own dying you must live, not mine.

It is my sincere hope that these ideas and practices will assist you, as they have me, to reveal and open some previously closed doors. Living our dying is the work of a lifetime. It is one way I know for us to actualize the greater work that is our life's birthright. Godspeed, my friend and fellow traveler.

This moment, here and now, is a beginning.

Dying is a beginning.

Afterword

Seek, keep seeking . . . So this is the end!
And it's nothing . . .

—TOLSTOY'S LAST WORDS

After reading an earlier draft of this book, a friend of mine asked, "If you could choose one moment from your life to live over again, what would it be?" What moment? What event? The remembrance that sprang to mind surprised me. I hadn't thought about it in years. If I could choose one moment to live again . . .

It would be the first time a group of us consciously came together to form a healing circle around a dying friend. The moment begins with James' eighty-something-pound body, looking like an Auschwitz victim, lying on the floor, tucked gently into pillows. The "Alleluia" chant playing softly in the candle-lit room. At least a dozen of us encircled around him. Palms outstretched, laid upon him. Not knowing whether to wish for a dramatic physical healing or a healing into a quicker death. Looking back and forth from James' face—his eyes mostly shut, slivers of white flickering between his lids, in ecstasy—looking back and forth from him to those of us joined around his frail body. Back and forth into our own eyes, some in wonder, others with tears rolling off their cheeks, heads bent over this frail, frail body. And Michael cradling, caressing James' head. A tear falling from Michael's face, landing on my hand, my bare hand laid upon James' chest. Heads bent, faces lowered. Like ancient monks, praying a long-practiced secret ritual. Heads bowed in awe of God. And over James. Kneeling at the altar. Beside James' body. Hands in prayer. Laid upon James' skin. Guinevere, Mark, Bill, Adrienne, Michael, Monty, Barry, Martin, Theo, Lundi, Steven, Delman—all of us singing "alleluia, alleluia, alleluia . . ." Not knowing what to wish for. Opening our hearts. Looking up from James to one another. Choreography by God. A dance around this healing into death. Fear. Opening. A moment in, a moment out. Of song, of love, of breath.

Yes, I'd rest myself in that moment if I could. Where I was big enough to contain my fear, my uncertainty, all of it, and still feel God and James and myself. I'd rest myself where there's no paradox in not knowing, where we join together, chanting and not knowing and crying and blessing and touching and deepening and singing, "Alleluia, alleluia." That's my moment. I'd rest right there and live it again and again, becoming as big as I can.

The fruit of living our dying is not only to be alive and awake to ourselves as we die, but to be alive and awake to ourselves and others as we live, too. An intimacy with all things. This intimacy begins and ends with ourselves, with a self-honesty toward what we're experiencing. It is the alpha and the omega.

In the "Preface," I asked the basic question: Why bother to live our dying? Why should we take the time and energy to do the emotional and spiritual work of consciously living our dying? There's not a simple answer. In a manner, this entire book is my attempt to answer that question. Perhaps, at this point along the way, you can understand for yourself why you must bother. It is still my prayer that you do, that you bother, too.

As I finish this collection of personal notes and remembrances, I feel a sense of incompleteness and loss. I feel loss because it's time to say good-bye, to let go of this sharing. Another death approaches. My feelings about incompleteness are not so obvious to me. I know it has something to do with intimacy.

At the point you're reading this now, this book has been through a long process of rewriting, with much of the accidental sloppiness removed. I hope its intimacy, its soul, remains intact. Because though its form is a book—in a way, a "how to" guide—in its soul, its heart, *Living Our Dying* is a love letter. If you decide to reread any of it, in whole or just a few pages, know that it's a love letter to each of us who seeks to live our dying. Though disguised as something more public and less intimate, I hope its heart betrays its true intentions.

Now, to completion. Just as part of me doesn't want to end this writing, another part of me knows it's time. Perhaps that is what the moment of death will be like, another part of us knowing it's time to move on. What was it the last chapter concludes with?—"Dying is a beginning."

But it still hurts at times. And we still want to run away at times. Our courage is in openly, honestly feeling the hurt, coming back into the sacred paradox of impermanence and God's grace both here, together, as one inseparable moment.

I honor you, my fellow traveler, for your own journey—for living our dying. And it is "our" dying. No one is an island here.

Godspeed . . .

With love,

Joseph

Arpin, Robert L. *Wonderfully, Fearfully Made*. New York:
   HarperCollins, 1993.
   An autobiography composed of a collection of letters by
   a gay Catholic priest with AIDS. I have often
   recommend this book to people who are dealing with issues
   concerning traditional Christianity, "God," and AIDS.

The Enlightened Heart. Edited by Stephen Mitchell. New York:
   HarperCollins, 1989.
   The best, most concise anthology of sacred poetry I've ever
   encountered. Sublime, simple, and something to be
   savored again and again. For those interested, Mitchell has
   compiled a companion volume of sacred prose, *The
   Enlightened Mind*.

Levine, Stephen. *Who Dies?: An Investigation of Conscious
   Living and Conscious Dying*. New York: Doubleday,
   1982; and *Healing Into Life and Death*. New York:
   Doubleday, 1987.
   If I had to choose a "must read" it would be these two
   books by Stephen Levine. *Who Dies* came first
   chronologically, so one might as well start there. Together
   they invite the reader, with forthright practices of

guided meditations, to enter deeply into the world of conscious dying. Filled with personal stories, guided meditations, and profound heart and insight. Stephen Levine is the author of several other books, all of them dealing with conscious living and dying in some way.

Lewis, C. S. *A Grief Observed*. New York: Harper and Row, 1952.

A brief and moving self-portrait of one of the twentieth century's authentic Christian apologists, who allows himself the honest process of grief, anger, and sincere religious questioning in light of his spouse's death. The book chronicles a greater healing as Lewis finds the courage to press his theology through an experiential real-life filter and see what emerges. I also suggest the movie *Shadowlands* (1993), which is a superb dramatic presentation of the story leading up to Lewis' insights.

Moore, Thomas. *Care of the Soul*. New York: HarperCollins, 1992.

Though not overtly about conscious dying, this book invites us into the deeper waters of conscious living. An exploration into the archetypal, mythological plane of our reality, examining how our wounds and shadows offer a way into a more whole experience of life and self.

Ram Dass and Paul Gorman. *How Can I Help?* New York: Knopf, 1991.

This is my suggested entry for anyone interested in "service" as a path for emotional and spiritual awakening. For professional care providers, this book is a must-read. Filled with stories and reflections, it is more literary than how-to-ish, addressing the heart and soul as well as the mind. A sampling of chapter titles: "Natural Compassion," "Who's Helping?," "Suffering," "The Listening Mind," "The Way of Social Action," "Burnout."

Schneider, David. *Street Zen: The Life and Work of Issan Dorsey.* Boston: Shambhala, 1993.
A biography of an American Zen priest's outrageous life. Dorsey founded San Francisco's Maitri Hospice. As a friend of mine says, "At the beginning of the book you're angry because he seems like such a pig, and by the end, you're crying because he's dying and you'll never get to meet him. Reading this book was a dying process for me: my judgments about spiritual correctness died and someone I had grown to care about, Issan, died too."